MS
SURGERY
5

Master Ser

Series Editor:
Dana K. Andersen, MD

Brought to you as an educational service by **MERCK**

Advance *noun*...progress, improvement, movement toward a goal.

Each volume in the Master Series in Surgery *will provide a comprehensive review of current advances in a major area of surgery. The objective is to provide the reader with practical, up-to-date information and to favor the clinical more than the experimental aspect of the topics presented. However, special attention will be devoted to the discussion of recent investigative findings that might impact the conduct of surgical and clinical practices in these areas. The volumes of the series are not intended to serve as "how-to" books, but as useful references by authorities in the field.*

Series Editor: Dana K. Andersen, MD

Forthcoming Volume:

Volume 6 Advances in Surgical Gene Therapy

Advances in Surgical Critical Care

Volume 5
Master Series in Surgery

Series Editor: Dana K. Andersen, MD
Professor of Surgery
Chief, Surgical Gastroenterology
Yale University School of Medicine

World Medical Press

Library of Congress Cataloging in Publication Data
Main entry under title:
Advances in Surgical Critical Care
(Master Series in Surgery)
Includes bibliographies and index.

Printed in the United States of America

ISBN 0-933751-08-7 World Medical Press

Preface

TO VOLUME 5

The critically ill or injured patient requires the surgeon to bring to bear all of the tools and judgment at his or her command. Keeping the pulmonary system functional while avoiding gut bacterial translocation, or maintaining hemodynamic stability while preserving fluid and electrolyte balance is a common challenge in the intensive care unit. Despite decades of descriptive research on the effects of injury on the composition of the body as a whole, our ability to rescue patients from multisystem collapse and promote anabolic synthesis and repair of injured tissue remains an imperfect science.

This volume of the *Master Series in Surgery* focuses on the current understanding of the critical principles of critical care and describes the state of the art of our therapeutic strategies for metabolic support and the treatment of patients with infection. The newest information on the relationship between cytokine release and function on the overall response to illness or injury is also reviewed.

In the section on nutrition in critically ill patients, John C. Alverdy, MD, carefully clarifies the basic principles of nutritional support but also emphasizes the limitation of our current use of nutritional therapy. Although most surgeons now accept without question the concept that nutritional support is part of good management of the critically ill, a beneficial effect on survival or morbidity depends on many individual details of nutritional support therapy. Dr Alverdy draws our attention to key tissue-specific nutrients, the role of the gut, and the probable importance of hormonal regulation of metabolism as factors that need to be addressed. The route of feeding and the possibly critical role of cholecystokinin are outlined carefully, as is the increasingly important observation of the need to provide substrate into the gastrointestinal tract as early as possible. How early that support should start is also under examination in this discussion, as are the specific guidelines regarding the number of calories, composition of calories delivered, and parameters with which the surgeon should be familiar to assess the need for, and the results of, nutritional support. Finally, the specific dangers of overfeeding and the negative impact on survival of inappropriately enthusiastic nutrient administration is described. The principles outlined in this section should guide surgeons in their approach to metabolic support in critical care.

In the section on the treatment of patients with infectious diseases, William G. Cheadle, MD, and Julio A. Ramirez, MD, first review the basic principles regarding host defense against infection and multiple-organ failure, including the specific cellular components that provide resistance to infectious organisms. They carefully outline the specific distinguishing features of the various categories of infectious agents to remind us of the strategies for specific antimicrobial attack on invading organisms, and the biologic basis for the selection of antibiotic therapy. In addition, these authors review some of the enzymatic and chemical consequences of bacterial invasion, and remind us of the multifactorial role of cytokines, complement, and amines in the response to infection. But the major part of the section is a clear review of the principles that guide empiric and specific therapy for infections, and those factors that determine the rational choice of the type of antibiotic, the timing of antibiotic therapy, and the role of multi-agent treatment in serious surgical infections. The results of some of the recent trials of monoclonal antibodies directed against endotoxin are also reviewed in this section, and we are provided with the most balanced and up-to-date summary available on the probable role of these agents in patients with infections. Basic strategies in the approach to common surgical problems are reviewed, and the importance of your local hospital antibiogram is explained.

A common theme in recent studies on metabolic support and treatment of infections is the role of cytokines as agents that mediate the body's response to sepsis, stress, and shock. In the section on cytokine regulation of the host response to sepsis, Stephen F. Lowry, MD, and Steven E. Calvano, PhD, review what is currently understood of the cytokine mediator system. As the body defends itself against foreign cells and substances the immune response mechanism calls to action phagocytic cells as well as lymphocytes. The direction and modification of this response is choreographed by secretory products of the natural and acquired immune systems, which consist largely of proteins now called cytokines. The properties of cytokines as relatively low–molecular weight peptides or glycoproteins that bind to specific cell surface receptors to effect specific responses are reviewed in detail. The important cytokines involved in infectious disease are then delineated and described. Their origin, mechanism of action, and clinically recognizable effects are summarized, as are their likely physiologic and pathophysiologic roles in the setting of critical illness. The summary of specific cytokines is broken down into those produced by phagocytes and those synthesized predominantly by lymphocytes, and this delineation helps to establish the basis for therapeutic strategies designed to modify cytokine-mediated responses. There are a number of naturally occurring cytokine antagonists that may be helpful in the control of the response to infection. In addition, there is now a range of synthetically produced cytokine antagonists, including agents that modify the synthesis or release of cytokines or prevent the binding of cytokines to their specific receptors. Drs Lowry and Calvano review the recently performed studies in critically ill patients in which antagonists of tumor necrosis factor and interleukin-1 were examined as adjuvant agents that may be helpful for patients in septic shock. However, the authors also review the possible evidence that the interference of cytokine production may have adverse effects in some critically ill patients. The cytokine cascade has evolved as a sophisticated and complex defense mechanism whose hallmarks include many of the clinical signs and symptoms that we associate with critical illness. As we move forward to alter or prevent these signs of disaster we must not impair the body's defense mechanisms to react to invading cells. This up-to-date review of an emerging area provides the surgeon with the best prospective with which to judge the newest work in this field.

Our editors of the fifth volume of the *Master Series in Surgery* include the following experts in their fields:

John C. Alverdy, MD, is Associate Professor of Surgery at The University of Chicago, Pritzker School of Medicine, and Co-Director of the Surgical Critical Care Service. He is a recognized authority on the role of nutritional and metabolic support in critical illness and an established investigator in the role of the gut in host defense mechanisms.

William G. Cheadle, MD, is Associate Professor of Surgery at the University of Louisville, and Director of the Surgical Intensive Care Unit and the Associate Chief of Staff for Research at the Veterans Administration Medical Center, Louisville, Kentucky. He is an established investigator in the area of surgical infection and immune responses, and is an expert in the area of antibiotic therapy.

Stephen F. Lowry, MD, is Professor of Surgery at the Cornell University School of Medicine, and Director of the Laboratory of Surgical Metabolism at the New York Hospital–Cornell Medical Center. He has contributed to many of the fundamental observations in the role of cytokines in host defense mechanisms, and is an established investigator in the area of cytokine effects in cancer, burns, and sepsis.

Dana K. Andersen, MD

Contributors

Series Editor:

Dana K. Andersen, MD
Professor of Surgery
Chief, Surgical Gastroenterology
Yale University School of Medicine

Volume Editors:

John C. Alverdy, MD
Associate Professor of Surgery
Co-Director, Surgical Critical Care Service
The University of Chicago
Pritzker School of Medicine

William G. Cheadle, MD
Associate Professor of Surgery
University of Louisville
Director, Surgical Intensive Care Unit
Associate Chief of Staff for Research
Veterans Administration Medical Center
Louisville, Kentucky

Stephen F. Lowry, MD
Professor of Surgery
Cornell University School of Medicine
Director, Laboratory of Surgical Metabolism
New York Hospital–Cornell Medical Center

Contents

I Nutrition in Critically Ill Patients

John C. Alverdy, MD

BRIEF CONTENTS

INTRODUCTION

Optimal Nutritional Support

Feed a cold, starve a fever. Or is it feed a fever, starve a cold? Historically, therapeutic starvation was a commonly accepted approach to the management of patients with fever and life-threatening illnesses. However, with the development of sophisticated methods of assessing energy and nutrient expenditure, it became clear that such patients were experiencing an increased breakdown of protein that could not be counterbalanced by consumption of the customary levels of nutrients. This knowledge, coupled with the availability of fluids permitting hyperalimentation (particularly intravenous nutrition), resulted in the ability to deliver more calories and protein than had ever been delivered to the critically ill. As the hazards of overfeeding were documented a moderate approach emerged. The elucidation of the metabolic consequences of stress and its mediation by various cytokine and endocrine pathways has raised the possibility that tissue-specific fuels, combined with hormonal and cytokine manipulation, may offer a novel means of maintaining and restoring organ function in the critically ill.

A brief history of nutritional support

How then do we determine optimal nutritional support? Traditionally, clinicians have used measures of lean body mass, nitrogen economy, and energy expenditure as their guides. Yet, while it is generally presumed that critically ill patients benefit from nutritional support, direct evidence for this observation remains elusive.[1] Few studies have documented that weight gain and nitrogen conservation alone are predictive of good outcome. Furthermore, are the clinical manifestations of the anabolic effects of exogenous calorie and nitrogen provision a result of the abatement of the underlying catabolic stress or a result of aggressive nutritional support? Most likely, the answer is both. It seems that attenuation of the cytokine response that mediates nitrogen wasting, in combination with tissue-specific nutrition, is required to influence outcome.

Problems in determining optimal nutrition

Attempts to achieve a positive nitrogen balance within 48 hours of injury or infection have been futile, resulting in excess caloric infusion, hyperglycemia, lipidemia, and abnormal hepatic function. Animal studies have demonstrated not only that weight gain and a positive nitrogen balance are exceedingly difficult to achieve during this time, but that they may not influence outcome. Thus, it is neither practical nor possible in many circumstances to override the catabolic effects of stress with currently available nutritional formulas. Further insight into this problem can be gained by examining the metabolic response to stress.

THE METABOLIC RESPONSE TO STRESS

Which Nutrients Are Expended?

Hypermetabolism, which is secondary to the release of the counterregulatory hormones, epinephrine, glucagon, and cortisol, accelerates protein breakdown and increases gluconeogenesis.[2] Infection, trauma, cancer, and other forms of inflammation activate the immune system through the production of highly potent molecules that are able to kill pathogens, destroy

Hypermetabolism and catabolism

aberrant cells, and increase nutrient uptake to stressed cells. Cytokines comprise the interleukins 1 through 12. Other mediators of importance include tumor necrosis factor (TNF) and the interferons. There is a significant interdependence between the neuroendocrine axis and the cytokine mediator system.[3] Amplification or attenuation of the stress response can be achieved through a complex network of paracrine, neurocrine, and endocrine signals (Fig. 1). Isotope determinations of substrate turnover have confirmed that, despite nutritional support in the critically ill, these catabolic influences persist.[4]

The cytokine-neuroendocrine axis

Figure 1

Although the mechanisms that mediate anabolic failure in the critically ill nutritionally supported patient are complex, it has become increasing clear that classical hormonal influences as well as cytokines contribute to this process. Therefore, asking to what extent nutritional support can influence outcome may really be asking how current nutrient formulations effect neuroendocrine and cytokine pathways. In reparable, limited-duration injuries the hormonal/cytokine response may promote the mobilization of endogenous energy sources and promote organ health. However, during periods of excessive stress hormone release and persistent cytokine production, prolonged injury may exhaust existing metabolic and immunologic reserves. While the current thinking is that nutritional support prevents this erosion of cell function, studies suggest that, under certain conditions, excessive or inappropriate nutritional support may "fuel the fire."[5]

Nutritional support effects cytokine and endocrine pathways

As the complex networks and signals in cells become better characterized, multiple techniques for blocking these effects will emerge. The most compelling arguments attesting to the importance of cytokines in the metabolic response come from studies in which cytokine production or receptor activation is blocked. These techniques use monoclonal antibodies and, in some cases, selective gene knockout to implicate a particular cytokine in the

Cytokines and the metabolic response to injury and infection

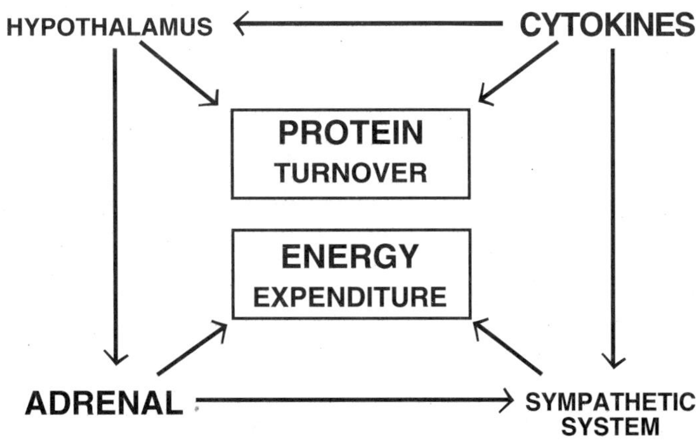

Fig.1. The network of paracrine, neurocrine, and endocrine signals through which amplification or attenuation of the stress response can be achieved.

hypermetabolic response to injury or infection.[6] Animal models that employ such blockade are associated with a diminished counterregulatory hormonal response, better nitrogen retention, and improved survival. Future approaches to the critically ill patient may involve the use of pharmacologic additives that attenuate protein erosion, permitting an adequate incorporation of calories and nitrogen into host cells. A better understanding of the regulatory pathways responsible for the metabolic response to injury will provide a unique opportunity for the development of more physiologic approaches to this complex problem.

The magnitude and duration of the metabolic response to injury and infection significantly influences the degree of hypermetabolism and immunosuppression. If attempts can be made to attenuate this response, there may be a recovery from postinjury immune dysfunction. Clinicians often face a frustrating lack of positive outcomes despite aggressive nutritional support.

Hyperalimentation solutions lack key nutrients and peptides

Table 1

Current hypotheses suggest that available hyperalimentation solutions are deficient in key tissue-specific nutrients and bioactive peptides that have been shown experimentally to attenuate the metabolic response to injury and improve outcome (Table 1). Furthermore, the lack of enteral stimulation by foodstuffs is an inherent flaw of intravenous nutrition; thus, it is not surprising that the capacity of nutritional support to maintain lean body mass and immune function during periods of maximal catabolic stress is limited. The provision of excess calories and nitrogen during these periods is insufficient to overcome the associated immune dysfunction and loss of lean tissue mass. Recognizing the limitations of current nutritional support formulas will permit the clinician to develop a rationale for deciding on the route of feeding, timing of nutritional support, and provision of key nutrients that may deliver tissue-specific substrates during periods of organ dysfunction.

ISSUES OF NUTRITIONAL SUPPORT

Route of Feeding

Enteral nutrition vs parenteral nutrition

Current experimental and clinical data favor the use of early enteral nutrition over parenteral nutrient infusion in the critically ill. Practice patterns in the United States of America have

Table 1.
Nutrients Lacking or in Low Quantity in Current Solutions

Amino Acids	Bioactive Peptides
Glutamine	β Casomorphine
Tyrosine	Polyamines
Cysteine	Spermine
Taurine	Dipeptides
Histidine	

demonstrated the popularity of early enteral access and the initiation of feeding within the first 24 hours of injury. This can be achieved with nasoenteric intubation, surgically placed feeding jejunal tubes, or endoscopically placed gastric tubes. Experience with the early feeding of elemental diets has demonstrated the feasibility of immediate poststress feeding, ileus notwithstanding.[7] Early enteral stimulation by foodstuffs is an attempt to maintain and restore the functional responsiveness of the intestinal barrier and immune system.

Disadvantages of parenteral nutrition

The administration of parenteral nutrition significantly compromises the intestinal barrier to bacteria and toxins.[8] The feeding of parenteral and oral elemental diets impairs mucosal immunoglobulin A (IgA) production, permits bacterial overgrowth of the indigenous coliform species, and allows increased permeation of luminal toxins (eg, endotoxin) and translocation of the facultative gram-negative bacteria to systemic organs, such as the liver, kidney, and mesenteric lymph nodes. Recently, the finding of altered intestinal permeability during total parenteral nutrition (TPN) has been observed in human volunteers.[9] Loss of epithelial barrier function between the intestinal lumen and the underlying vascular compartment can result in the absorption of proinflammatory macromolecules of limitless diversity. Intestinal hyperpermeability induced by TPN then may result in the activation of the same inflammatory mediators (cytokines) responsible for the catabolic stress response. Therefore, diets that do not maintain the normal function of the intestinal barrier may have counterproductive effects on host inflammation. While attempting to restore body composition during periods of negative nitrogen balance, the use of parenteral diets actually may impact negatively on outcome due to their quiescent effect on the intestinal immunologic barrier.

The emerging importance of the intestinal tract as an immune and metabolic organ has forced us to rethink the effects of diet on intestinal integrity and function. While the "disuse" effect of TPN on the intestinal tract has been well documented anatomically, no immediate deleterious consequences have been thought to occur.

Total parenteral nutrition impairs intestinal integrity and function

Total parenteral nutrition results in mucosal cell atrophy, diminution of the mucosal Ig response, decreased mucosal brush border enzyme activity, bacterial overgrowth, altered motility, and mucosal hyperpermeability. These effects are attenuated by the use of chemically defined enteral diets. The immediate consequence of these findings is that the transport of autotoxic macromolecules, which are ubiquitous in the intestinal lumen, may be concentrated within mucosal cells and stimulate the inflammatory pathways, which may be harmful to host recovery. For example, TNF is a multifunctional cytokine released by monocytes that mediates inflammation during periods of infection.

Hazards of TNF release during TPN

A study by Fong et al[10] found that human volunteers subjected to 7 days of TPN released increased amounts of TNF in response to an infectious stress, compared with enterally fed, age-matched subjects. Similar findings have been demonstrated in numerous animal studies in which rats given TPN were compared with rats nourished normally.[11] Of interest, the selective elimination of intestinal bacteria attenuates these results.[12] Therefore, it is possible that TPN alters the intestinal containment of the luminal flora and toxins such that an exaggerated inflammatory state results from an infectious or traumatic insult.

The production of numerous other cytokines and proinflammatory mediators is increased during parenteral feeding but their significance is unclear. However, it is possible to formulate a hypothesis to explain the adverse outcomes associated with TPN in patients experiencing severe and prolonged catabolic stress. Under conditions of appropriate enteral nutrition the intestinal barrier remains intact, and the systemic and local inflammatory cells are not exposed to the proinflammatory macromolecules that are present in the intestinal lumen. However, the use of TPN results in an impairment of this barrier, and local and remote cells of inflammation express an increased cytokine production. Because inflammation can occur without the detection of specific serum markers, organ dysfunction may occur and elude the clinician. This state of disordered inflammation may be driven by the inappropriate priming of the immune system from intestinal antigens.

Hypothesis concerning TPN and understimulation of the gut

The use of enteral stimulation by foodstuffs appears to maintain intestinal barrier mechanisms with much greater intensity and duration than does parenteral nutrition. In fact, the more complex the foodstuffs, the greater the stimulation of the intestinal immune and barrier activity. Rats nourished with whole protein are able to maintain barrier function more easily than are rats fed single–amino acid solutions. The use of bulking agents, such as nonnutritive fiber solutions, helps stimulate the mucosal adaptive response and attenuate TPN-induced alterations in barrier function. Diets with complex fats rather than short-chain fats also help maintain normal barrier function during periods of stress. The key to understanding these finding may be recognizing the importance of the effect of diet on the neuroendocrine immune system of the gut.

Effect of diet on the neuroendocrine-immune system of the gut

Foods that elicit strong endocrine responses from the intestine usually are complex foodstuffs. These responses include the release of cholecystokinin (CCK), neurotensin, substance P, and other neuropeptides. The importance of maintaining the normal activation and release of these brain/gut peptides following the ingestion of foodstuffs can be appreciated by recognizing their pleiotropic effects on a number of important organ systems. For example, normal amounts of CCK are released only after the infusion of whole protein into the duodenum; protein digests and amino acids have little effect.[13] Traditionally we think of CCK as a peptide that causes contraction of the gallbladder; however, its release is essential for lymphocyte function, intestinal motility, IgA production, and heart contractility.[14] Therefore, the neural, endocrine, and autocrine responses to luminal nutrition are important signals to remote tissues involved in circulatory, immunologic, and motor activities. Studies in which CCK activity is blocked have demonstrated significant impairment of these functional responses.[15] Following the ingestion of a CCK-stimulat-

Pleiotropic effects of peptides on organ systems

ing meal, splanchnic blood flow is increased by vasodilation of the splanchnic vascular bed and an increase in cardiac output. When human volunteers were administered a CCK receptor antagonist, attenuation of the postprandial increase in cardiac output was observed. It is known that heart muscle responds to CCK with an increase in contractility and rate.[16] Therefore, the attenuation of meal-induced CCK release may impair intestinal blood flow during periods of increased demand.

Total parenteral nutrition results in no CCK activity or release. Several adverse immune and hemodynamic consequences have been demonstrated with the administration of TPN but not the enteral presentation of nutrients. It is not yet known whether artificial nutrition affects the responses of other neuropeptides, such as neurotensin, which is important for gut blood flow, or substance P, which is an important neurotransmitter for a variety of organs. Food-induced neuroendocrine responses may be one way in which nutrients maintain the health of the host, not only by providing substrate for cell metabolism, but by eliciting paracrine and autocrine signals that stimulate remote cell functions. The bypassing of these signals with TPN or elemental diets may be an undesirable effect, the immediate consequences of which are just beginning to be recognized. Unfortunately, the clinician is often presented with the dichotomous task of using complex foodstuffs to stimulate gut function in patients whose gastrointestinal tracts are incapable of tolerating such forms of alimentation. This situation has been the main impetus for the development of nutrient formulas that are absorbed completely yet provide bowel rest.

A local food-induced neuroendocrine response in maintaining systemic health

Recognizing the need for enteral stimulation by more complex foods has resulted in several novel approaches to this problem. Combined enteral and parenteral alimentation, elemental feeding with fiber supplementation, and the use of parenteral/elemental diets in conjunction with CCK infusion have been tried. Peptide-based diets that are nonelemental in form stimulate gut blood flow, increase immune function, and are readily absorbed. The use of short-chain fatty acids and glutamine-rich diets also may activate immune function directly and indirectly. Total parenteral nutrition solutions administered with bolus infusions of CCK improve intestinal barrier function and liver histology, and lower the incidence of acalculous cholecystitis.[17] Total parenteral nutrition solutions supplemented with neurotensin attenuate changes in intestinal permeability and are trophic to the intestinal mucosa.[18] Therefore, one emerging approach to counteract the quiescent effect of artificial nutrition on the intestinal neuroendocrine response is the use of bioactive mimicry to reproduce these effects. As a better understanding of the influences of food on the neuroendocrine immune system evolves, hospital diets that stimulate this system more physiologically will be developed.

Peptide-based diets

Supplemented TPN solutions

Timing of Nutritional Support

One specific issue regarding nutritional support in the critically ill patient is the timing of early nutritional intervention. The

"Early" nutritional support

question remains, how early is *early*? While clinicians have always recognized the relationship between progressive malnutrition and susceptibility to infection, the precise determination of the timing of nutritional therapy has remained a subject of much debate. During periods of hemodynamic instability or multiple surgical interventions, the use of continuous enteral or parenteral feeding is often impractical. Most studies define "early" nutritional support as that which is begun within 48 hours of hospital admission. The goal of early feeding must not override stabilization of the patient's hemodynamic, electrolyte, and acid-base status.

Most critically ill patients develop ileus, which can limit the ability of the gastrointestinal tract to tolerate adequate feedings. Postoperative ileus usually is confined to the stomach and colon. In fact, intact peristalsis in the small bowel is usually observed at the conclusion of major intestinal surgery. One method of assessing small-bowel viability following resection is to manually stimulate the bowel and observe coordinated peristalsis. Because of these observations, the use of techniques to establish enteral access into the small intestine have become popular. These include needle-catheter jejunostomies, the nasoenteric placement of feeding tubes, and Roux-en-Y feeding jejunostomies. These techniques establish access for immediate feeding following surgery or admission to the hospital. The immediate postoperative administration of liquid diets is safe and can be initiated in the recovery room. Some surgeons have even begun small-bowel feeding during surgery to continually stimulate the mucosa and protect it from injury. However, these efforts may be excessive and have not gained popularity.

Establishing access to the small bowel for enteral feeding

Fewer septic complications with early enteral feeding

In humans there have been few studies demonstrating the benefits of early over late enteral nutrition. However, several well-designed, randomized, prospective studies have established that early enteral nutrition results in reduced septic complications in trauma patients.

The most recent study to document these effects was reported by Kudsk et al.[19] In 98 patients a needle-catheter jejunostomy was placed at the time of laparotomy. Patients were then randomized to receive enteral feeding or TPN, which was started within 24 hours of definitive abdominal surgery. The patients were followed until discharge, for 15 days, or until the occurrence of a septic complication, whichever came first. The investigators' goals were to achieve protein concentrations of 1.5 to 2 g/kg per day and nonprotein concentrations of 30 to 35 kcal/kg per day in each patient. They administered TPN to enterally fed patients only if 50% of these concentrations could not be achieved by day 7. Although the enterally fed patients received fewer nonprotein calories/kg per day than did the patients receiving TPN, they experienced significantly fewer septic complications. Particular benefit was noted in the more severely injured patients. Only two patients receiving enteral feeding were unable to attain 50% of their goal by day 7, and required TPN.

In addition to the reduced incidence of septic complications with early enteral feeding, nutrient effects on hepatic protein synthesis have been noted. Studies have demonstrated an increase in the concentrations of various constitutive proteins, such as albumin, prealbumin, transferrin, retinol-binding protein, and α_2-macroglobulin, during the course of 10 days in patients receiving enteral nutrition.[20] These values tended to decrease in TPN-fed patients.

Subsequently, Kudsk et al[21] showed that the reduction in acute phase protein production and hepatic reprioritization in the most severely injured patients was a result of the reduced septic complications that occurred in the enterally fed group, rather than a direct effect of enteral nutrition on liver protein synthesis. Only in patients with less severe injury did enteral feeding appear to have a beneficial effect on liver protein parameters.

Enteral feeding within 36 hours in humans

Grahm[22] randomized head-injured patients to early (within 36 hours) jejunal or delayed (following 3 to 5 days) gastric or jejunal feeding. Length of stay in the intensive care unit (ICU) and incidence of infectious complications were decreased significantly in the patients who were fed jejunally. Eyer[23] performed a similar study in which blunt trauma patients were randomized to receive early (within 24 hours) or late (following 72 hours) enteral feeding. There were no differences between the two groups as regards nitrogen balance, excretion of urinary catecholamines, serum cortisol levels, length of stay in the ICU, number of days on a ventilator, or individual infections. Thus, feeding within 72 hours of admission to a critical care unit is not universally accepted as beneficial.

Enteral feeding within 2 hours in animals

However, results of animal studies suggest that feeding within 2 hours of injury can attenuate the catabolic hormone response and the effects of stress on the intestinal barrier. Ostensibly, the rationale behind early enteral nutrition is the attenuation of the counterregulatory response and the relief of catabolic stress on the host. Although these findings have been well documented in animal studies, they have not been observed consistently in studies of heterogeneous patient populations in modern ICUs. Still, it appears reasonable to administer enteral nutrition within 72 hours of hospital admission, provided the patient is hemodynamically stable and the underlying problem may be treated definitively by surgery.

Enteral feeding within 72 hours seems reasonable

Nutrient Administration

Problems of determining caloric needs

Calories. Determining the best method for calculating the caloric needs of the critically ill patient remains a point of controversy. Numerous equations incorporating stress and activity factors have been developed. Unfortunately, recent studies suggest that these equations overestimate energy requirements by as much as 30%.[24]

Indirect calorimetry has received a great deal of attention, as portable devices have become less expensive and easy to calibrate. Their reliability and ease of use permits the direct measurement of oxygen consumption. While indirect calorimetry may accurately reflect energy requirements during a 20- to 30-minute period of equilibration, the practicality of its extrapolation to a 24-hour period remains unclear. Furthermore, while

Indirect calorimetry measurement by oxygen consumption

these machines are useful, they are costly, and no data have yet demonstrated improved patient outcome as a result of their use. Therefore, most studies suggest that, for the majority of critically ill patients, 25 to 30 cal/kg per day is a reasonable goal. In this case, the total caloric load of a 70-kg man would be 2,100 cal/d, which appears inadequate based on common practices of the last decade. However, exceeding this infusion rate of nonprotein calories appears to be associated with various manifestations of overfeeding. Furthermore, a growing body of evidence suggests that permissive underfeeding of the critically ill may be beneficial.

Goal of 25 to 30 cal/kg per day

Sources of Nonprotein Calories. The use of trimixture formulas has popularized the concept of the total nutrient admixture as a more physiologic and well-balanced method of TPN and enteral nutrition. The optimal rate of glucose infusion is approximately 4 mg/kg per minute. While glucose disposal in noncritically ill patients is traditionally between 5 and 7 mg/kg per minute, exceeding 4 mg/kg per minute results in excess calories being stored as body lipid rather than being oxidized. The clinical consequences of exceeding an infusion rate of 4 mg/kg per minute in the critically ill include cholestasis, steatosis, hypercarbia, and hyperosmolar states. Therefore, the addition of fat to constitute approximately 30% of the total nonprotein calories has become popular.

Glucose infusion rate

Fat emulsions may offer distinct advantages beyond the provision of essential fatty acids. They are a good source of dense calories (ie, less volume per gram of calorie), which is especially important in patients who require volume restriction, such as cardiac and renal failure patients. Fat emulsions also may have distinct advantages in patients who are dependent on mechanical ventilation. Because the respiratory quotient (CO_2 production/O_2 production) for fat is less than that for glucose, patients who have specific problems with hypercarbia may tolerate these mixed fuel sources better than they would glucose infusions alone. In addition, diabetics and patients receiving steroids may have better glucose control and reduced insulin requirements if they are given fat-based feeding formulas. Lessening the requirement for insulin is extremely helpful in patients whose sodium and volume requirements are limited.

Advantages to fat emulsion as a source of nonprotein calories

However, there are several disadvantages to fat emulsions. Studies suggest that the type as well as the quantity of fat can adversely affect immune function. Deficient fat intake results in the involution of lymphoid tissue, depressed antibody responses, and increased susceptibility to infection. Excess fat intake (especially the ingestion of long-chain fatty acids) decreases cell-mediated immunity, inhibits Ig synthesis, and depresses reticuloendothelial cell function.[25] These effects may be lessened with the ingestion of medium- or short-chain fatty acids. Also, the addition of omega-3 fatty acids may improve the immune response.[26]

Disadvantages to fat emulsion as a source of nonprotein calories

Current information suggests that an optimal method of providing nonprotein calories to the critically ill is to give them a mixture in which the carbohydrate:fat ratio is approximately

70:30 ratio of carbohydrate:fat

70:30. The advantages to using glucose solutions supplemented with periodic fat infusions include lower cost, anabolic effects due to insulin release, and long storage times. The critically ill patient should never receive more than 30% of his or her nonprotein calories as fat. The development of newer formulas with short- or medium-chain fatty acids may prove useful in specific disease states where their effects on the immune system are well established.

Determining protein requirements

Issues of Protein Quantity. Because the exact protein losses in the critically ill are difficult to measure, current practices are to assign a value of protein requirement based on body weight. Estimates of protein requirement in the critically ill range from 1 to 3 g/kg per day. The standard ratio of 150 cal/g nitrogen is generally accepted as optimal. Various modifications of this range have been developed for organ failure states or burn injury. Due to the catabolic effects of the metabolic response to injury, the utilization of exogenously provided protein for synthetic purposes plateaus at approximately 1.5 g/kg per day. The administration of protein above this level rarely contributes to the restoration of a positive nitrogen balance. However, the administration of up to 2 g protein/kg per day is reasonable in burn patients who are losing excess protein from the burn wound itself.

Issues of Protein Quality. The repeated observation that nitrogen balance remains negative in critically ill patients despite efforts of protein provision attests to the complex nature of feeding the critically ill. Current formulations of nutrients are based on the nutritional requirements of growing children and do not provide what are now considered conditionally essential nutrients. Traditionally, nutrient formulations have used inexpensive protein sources and filler amino acids to meet the needs of catabolic patients. It was assumed that if the traditionally essential amino acids were available, the nonessential amino acids could be synthesized de novo. The concept of conditionally essential amino acids—nonessential amino acids that cannot be synthesized from essential amino acids during critical illness—has led to a rethinking of current formulas for nutritional support. Glutamine, the preferred respiratory fuel for the small intestine, is lacking in all TPN solutions and many enteral formulas. Because the catabolic response to stress impairs the synthesis and utilization of this amino acid, patients who are alimented for prolonged periods with glutamine-free solutions become glutamine deficient.[27] This also may be true for other conditionally essential, high-biologic–priority amino acids, such as tyrosine and arginine. Therefore, one hypothesis currently being tested is whether the infusion of high biologic proteins can attenuate the negative nitrogen balance that occurs at times of catabolic stress in critically ill patients.

Rethinking current formulas for nutritional support

For many reasons, current methods of alimentation in the critically ill do not attenuate the counterregulatory responses and negative nitrogen balance inherent in this population. Most obvious is the fact that critically ill patients are often paralyzed or deeply sedated; therefore, exogenous nitrogen sources cannot

Factors in negative nitrogen balance

be incorporated into inactive muscle sites. Strategies such as intermittent exercise (using periods of decreased ventilatory support and oscillating beds) will increase muscle demand and uptake into cells. Even the application of electrical stimulation to enhance the contraction of selected muscles has been attempted. A final approach involves the use of growth hormone (GH).

Amino acid imbalances in hyperalimentation solutions

Another possible factor contributing to the negative nitrogen balance of the critically ill is the imbalance of amino acids in hyperalimentation solutions. It is also possible that intravenous and enteral formulas should be peptide-based rather than single amino acid–based. Studies that have examined amino acid fluxes in skeletal muscle suggest that essential amino acids, branch-chain amino acids, glutamine, and arginine are mobilized at high rates. One would then assume that solutions formulated to reflect these effluxes would result in nitrogen conservation. Yet, little enhancement of the protein synthetic potential has been demonstrated with some of these designer formulas. This may be due to the fact that the counterregulatory response to stress prefers endogenous sources of protein to exogenous sources, and that a more rational approach is to pharmacologically manipulate the response and provide formulas that are well utilized under these circumstances. For example, arginine may be important to the diet, and high concentrations of arginine, provided in some formulas, are thought to elicit some of their effects by stimulating GH secretion. However, the use of high-arginine diets may be overshadowed by the administration of GH, which is associated with higher plasma concentrations than is arginine. In this way, certain nutrients can act as drugs and certain drugs can influence nutrient utilization. For these reasons, future strategies for nutritional support of the critically ill will likely involve a multimodality approach to conserve nitrogen.

MONITORING NUTRITIONAL SUPPORT

Laboratory Tests or Functional End Points?

The elegant work of Jeejeebhoy during the last decade has led us to question the validity of increasing lean body mass and weight gain as appropriate measures of adequate nutritional support. Lean body mass consists of water, potassium, nitrogen, and glycogen. Recent studies have shown that malnutrition and refeeding alter total body potassium concentrations earlier than, and differently from the way in which, they alter total body nitrogen levels. These findings suggest than an early effect of nutrition occurs with membrane ion transport. In support of this concept, Jeejeebhoy and others have found that nutrition alters muscle performance earlier than it alters body composition. In addition, changes in muscle function correlate with surgical outcomes. Loss of body protein alone without altered performance does not correlate with complications in surgical patients. Therefore, starvation and its associated changes in body mass is not the same as malnutrition, where function changes in organ performance are demonstrated. For example, muscle and skeleton size in adults are dependent on exercise and gravity. Astronauts lose calcium and develop muscular atrophy. This is

Membrane ion transport

The difference between starvation and malnutrition

similar to the situation of patients who are bedridden and ventilator-dependent. Their weight loss and reduced muscle size do not indicate malnutrition but, rather, disuse atrophy. Also, diseases resulting in protein loss from the gut as a result of inflammation can decrease serum protein concentrations while nutrient intake is normal. Therefore, bedside anthropometric measurements, plasma protein profiles, and alterations in immune competence that result from the underlying disease process itself may not be valid indications of malnutrition or efficacy of current nutritional support.

Measuring body composition directly

Newer techniques have been developed to measure body composition directly, to determine whether there is a correlation between lean tissue or fat and nutritional outcome. When a high-frequency alternating current is passed through the body there is a total opposition to current flow called impedance, which can be resolved into a resistive component and a reactive component. The resistance depends on the body's water and ion content. Because total body water is a combination of extracellular and intracellular fluids, bioelectrical impedance analysis is an index of lean body mass (intracellular fluids) and extracellular fluid. This technique consists of placing aluminum foil spot electrodes on the dorsal surfaces of the hands and feet. An excitation current of 800 mA at 50 kHz is introduced and resistance is determined. Measurements are performed on both sides of the body, and the lowest resistance value is recorded. Although this instrumentation is available only at specialized centers, it offers a method of establishing the validity of body composition measurement as a way of predicting nutrient efficacy. When these studies are correlated to muscle function parameters, such as force frequency curves or muscle relaxation rates, a lack of correlation is seen between changes in measures of lean body mass and muscle function. The endurance properties of important muscle beds may not depend on the loss or restoration of lean body mass. Therefore, failure to achieve positive nitrogen balance or weight gain in the critically ill patient should not discourage the clinician and lead him or her to believe that nutritional support is inefficacious or inadequate.

Monitoring nutritional support

Monitoring the nutritional progress of the critically ill includes performing a subjective global assessment, obtaining a nutritional history, performing a physical examination, and treating the underlying disorder while minimizing periods of inanition. Using conventional measures of nutrient efficacy, such as nitrogen balance, weight gain, and visceral protein markers during the first 72 hours play little role in the monitoring of nutritional support. Once the hypermetabolic response to stress has abated a more routine use of these markers during the patient's nutritional rehabilitation may be helpful.

THE DELETERIOUS EFFECTS OF OVERFEEDING

Overfeeding involves the administration of calories or protein in excess of specific needs. However, because specific disease states and patient age, weight, gender, and height vary according to clinical circumstances, it is often difficult to determine when a

Table 2

patient is being overfed. The potential hazards of overfeeding are listed in Table 2; their risk is greatest in the very young, very old, and those most severely stressed.

Stress-induced hypermetabolism cannot be reversed by overfeeding as long as there is a persistence of the hormonal/cytokine alterations causing the stress. In fact, excess calories actually may increase hepatic workload and the hypermetabolic response to injury. Additionally, hepatic compromise due to overfeeding in the absence of stress may decrease hepatic metabolic function in response to a subsequent stress, especially an infectious stress. One study in which rats were overfed enterally or fed normally before being subjected to cecal ligation and puncture showed marked decreases in hepatic protein and synthesis rates in the normally fed animals. Further, hepatomegaly was more prominent and amount of liver protein/g of tissue significantly lower in the overfed animals than in the normally fed animals. It is particularly important to recognize that overfeeding-induced changes in liver function are not always accompanied by morphologic changes, and that these effects are exaggerated during periods of infectious stress.

Overfeeding-induced changes in liver function

Because overfeeding has been associated with significant alterations in immune function it is logical to assume that it would lead to decreased survival in patients. Although studies have provided compelling proof that overfeeding does decrease survival in animals, few data are available in humans, although the effect of caloric overfeeding with high-carbohydrate infusions was studied in postoperative adults. Vo et al[28] randomized patients to receive a high-calorie diet or a low-calorie diet. The patients who were placed on the high-calorie diet received 150% of measured energy expenditure whereas the patients who were placed on the low-calorie diet received 100% of measured energy expenditure. Mortality was significantly greater in the patients receiving the high-calorie diet than in those receiving the low-calorie diet (40% vs 28%; $P < 0.05$).

Overfeeding and increased mortality in clinical studies

An animal study using an established model of burn wound sepsis stratified guinea pigs by varying degrees of caloric intake (100, 125, 150, or 175 kcal/kg per day).[29] Decreased survival was observed in animals fed 150 and 175 kcal/kg per day (mortality, 100% in both groups) compared with animals fed 125 kcal/kg per

Overfeeding and decreased survival in animal studies

Table 2. Potential Hazards of Overfeeding
Hyperglycemia
Hypertriglyceridemia
Respiratory insufficiency
Electrolyte disorder
Abnormal liver function
Azotemia
Immunosuppression

day (mortality, 62.5%) or 100 kcal/kg per day (mortality, 42.8%). Of note, 175 kcal/kg per day is estimated to be the optimal caloric load for guinea pigs subjected to burn wound sepsis. The lack of a positive outcome despite this "optimal" nutritional intake underscores the complex undertaking of appropriate nutritional support in the critically ill.

Adverse effects of overfeeding on survival during infection in animals

A final important point is that overfeeding during a prestress period will have a significant adverse effect on outcome should a subsequent infectious insult occur. In another study, acute bacterial peritonitis was induced in rats fed normally for 6 days or overfed for 6 days. The overfed rats demonstrated a mortality of 53% compared with the normally fed rats, who demonstrated a mortality of 14%.[30] Thus, precise protein-calorie support during the entire period of alimentation is important even if the hypermetabolic response to stress has abated.

THE BENEFICIAL EFFECTS OF PERMISSIVE UNDERFEEDING

Although growth curves appear optimal during ad libitum feeding, longevity in overfed animals is decreased compared with that in calorie- or protein-restricted animals. In a study by Nolen,[31] rats were fed ad libitum or given a diet that restricted their calorie and protein intake by 20% or 40%. The animals given the restricted diets had retarded growth curves and grew to be smaller adults. However, they remained healthier than did the rats fed ad libitum, and lived longer (average longevity, 856 days in the rats on the 20% restricted diet; 924 days in the rats on the 40% restricted diet; and 706 days in the rats fed ad libitum). Similar studies have been performed by Berg and Simms,[32] who reported significant increases in longevity (average longevity, 1,005 days in male rats on a restricted diet; 802 days in male rats fed ad libitum; 1,294 days in female rats on a restricted diet; and 930 days in female rats fed ad libitum). Further, disease onset was delayed in the diet-restricted animals. Ross also reported a lower mortality among animals receiving protein-restricted diets.

Permissive underfeeding favors longevity in animal studies

This recurring discrepancy between changes in body composition and clinical outcome as a result of age, stress, or infection continues to challenge the conventional wisdom of increasing caloric/protein intake. Even severe protein/calorie deprivation impairs growth, depresses immune function, and increases susceptibility to infection and stress. Although restricting dietary intake to a level that sustains suboptimal growth but increases immune function and survival may seen dichotomous, it may prove to be a rational approach to the critically ill patient. Certainly the overfeeding of the critically ill is unwarranted. However, permissive underfeeding may actually improve survival more than "normal" feeding for a patient with a given disease state.

Restricted dietary intake: A rational approach?

As mentioned above, the results of studies in guinea pigs subjected to burn injury suggest that feeding 20% less than "appropriate" increases survival in models of chronic lethal sepsis. While the literature is replete with reports of the effects of calorie restriction on immune function, the findings appear conflicting. Severe protein/calorie deprivation impairs immune function whereas moderate deprivation improves immunity. The question now is whether sufficient information is available for the clinician to navigate the difficult course of providing "adequate" nutrition or "lesser" nutrition without falling below the threshold of clearly "inadequate" nutrition. Because every patient's nutritional requirements depend on a variety of factors, we must temper our zeal for permissive underfeeding until more clinical information is available.

Hypothesis: Patients are not adapted to aggressive ICU nutritional support

An interesting hypothesis for the beneficial effects of permissive underfeeding is that the human immune system has not yet fully adapted to the current life support systems used in ICUs. Evolutionary pressures have selected for adaptive responses that are characterized by anorexia, fever, and reduced nutrient intake. Most highly evolved mammals do not have support systems to take over breathing, eating, and circulatory support during periods of illness. Modern intensive care therapy is only 25 years old. During periods of critical illness from prehistoric times to the recent past the normal adaptive response to injury involved the limited availability of food. The adaptive response to injury and inanition may limit feeding-induced cytokine production and the generation of inflammatory pathways from substrates that will produce harmful agents and tissue injury. The approach of aggressive feeding during the early phases of injury may be premature in view of the lack of time for evolutionary pressure to adapt humans to life-saving intensive care therapies. Short-term undernutrition then may prove to be beneficial during periods of intense systemic inflammation and improve overall survival.

ADJUNCTIVE HORMONAL THERAPY DURING NUTRITIONAL SUPPORT

Growth Hormone and Insulin-Like Growth Factor

Anabolic effects of growth hormone

Table 3

The anabolic effects of GH had been documented as early as the 1950s when pituitary-derived extracts were administered to critically ill burn patients.[33] In several studies GH therapy has improved nitrogen balance even better than have hypocaloric diets.[34] The degree of protein retention is substantial when determined over a 2-week course of critical illness. The beneficial effects of GH occur in an anabolic hormonal milieu induced by the administration of the hormone because plasma levels of GH, insulin, and insulin-like growth factor (IGF)-I are consistently increased in a dose-related fashion (Table 3). These effects are regarded as functionally beneficial, as GH also has been shown to improve indices of skeletal muscle strength in stable postoperative patients and patents with chronic obstructive pulmonary disease.[35,36]

The effects of insulin-like growth factor–I

The mechanisms by which the exogenous administration of GH effects protein economy are multifactorial but are believed to be mediated by the endogenous production of IGF-I,[37] which has insulin-like effects on fat, carbohydrates, and protein metabolism, and is believed to be responsible for most of the anabolic effects of GH. In animal studies, GH treatment increased the synthesis of IGF-I by the liver, its major site of production. The administration

**Table 3.
Possible Mechanisms for the Effect of Growth Hormone on Protein Metabolism**

Reduced amino acid efflux
Maintenance of intracellular glutamine concentration
Increased blood growth hormone, insulin-like growth factor–I, and insulin concentrations
Maintenance of cellular water compartment
Enhanced fat oxidation and increased serum free fatty acids

of recombinant IGF-I itself has been shown to induce anabolic effects in normally fed and hypocalorically fed subjects.[38]

Studies in animals and humans have demonstrated that GH and IGF-I administration increase protein-rich tissue even during periods of hypocaloric feeding. It can be reasoned that the current approach of feeding calories to meet specific needs at times when the metabolic response prevents the use of exogenous nutrients in critically ill, catabolic, weight-losing patients may not achieve the best results. Future research that defines the role of anabolic agents or agents that attenuate the catabolic response may permit the use of feeding regimens that are well tolerated during critical illness. A better understanding of the mechanisms of the actions and limitations of current formulas of nutritional support for the critically ill will pave the way for more physiologic strategies for dealing with the catabolic stress of critical illness.

Future trends

References

1. Herndon DN, et al. *J Trauma* 1987;27:195-204.
2. Kinney J. *Acta Chir Scand* 1984;522(suppl):45-56.
3. Barber A. *Surg Forum* 1990;41:74-77.
4. Moller-Loswick AC, et al. *JPEN* 1991;15:669-675.
5. Coyle SM, et al. *Clin Nutr* 1990;9:20.
6. Tracey KJ, et al. *Nature* 1987;330:662-664.
7. Moore EE, et al. *J Trauma* 1986;26:874-881.
8. Burke D, et al. *Arch Surg* 1989;124:1396-1399.
9. Buchman AL, et al. *Gastroenterology* 1993;104:A612.
10. Fong Y, et al. *Ann Surg* 1989;210:449.
11. Saito H, et al. *JPEN* 1987;11:1.
12. Offenbartl K, et al. *Surg Res Comm* 1989;46:46.
13. Sharara AI, et al. *Am J Physiol* 1993;265:28.
14. Stead RH, et al. *Immunol Rev* 1987;100:333.
15. Freier S, et al. *Gastroenterology* 1987;93:1242.
16. Fiedorowicz RJ. *Pol J Pharmacol Pharm* 1989;41:561-572.
17. Curran TJ, et al. *Surg Forum* 1993;44:638-641.
18. Helton WS, et al. *Gastroenterology* 1991;100:A525.
19. Kudsk KA, et al. *Ann Surg* 1992;215:503-513.
20. Peterson VM, et al. *Surgery* 1988;104:199-207.
21. Kudsk KA, et al. *ASPEN Conference Symposium*, Orlando, Florida, Jan 19, 1992.
22. Grahm TW. *Neurosurgery* 1989;25:729-735.

23. Eyer SD. *J Trauma* 1993;34:639-644.
24. Bursztein S. *Acute Care* 1988;14:91-110.
25. Alexander JW, et al. *Ann Surg* 1986;204:1-8.
26. Daly JM, et al. *Surgery* 1992;112:56-67.
27. Abumrad NN. *Am J Physiol* 1989;257:E228-E234.
28. Vo NM, et al. *Am Surg* 1987;53:632-635.
29. Alexander JW, et al. *Ann Surg* 1989;209:334-340.
30. Yamazaki K. *J Surg Res* 1986;40:152-158.
31. Nolen GA. *J Nutr* 1972;102:1477-1494.
32. Berg BN, et al. *J Nutr* 1961;75:197-210.
33. Prudden JF, et al. *Surg Gynecol Obstet* 1956;102:695-701.
34. Liljedahl S, et al. *Acta Chir Scand* 1961;122:1-14.
35. Hammarqvist F, et al. *Ann Surg* 1992;216:184-191.
36. Vaara-Thorbeck R. *Hepatogastroenterology* 1992;39:270-274.
37. Kimbrough T. *J Surg Res* 1991;51:472-476.
38. Jiang ZM. *Ann Surg* 1989;210:513-524.

II Treatment of Infectious Disease

William G. Cheadle, MD
Julio A. Ramirez, MD

BRIEF CONTENTS

INTRODUCTION

Common surgical infections

Infection and multiple-organ dysfunction or failure are the most common causes of late death following trauma. Infections commonly noted in the surgical intensive care unit (SICU) include major wound infections, such as necrotizing fasciitis; nosocomial infections, such as nosocomial pneumonia; fungal infections; urinary tract infections; intra-abdominal infections; and intravascular catheter-related infections.[1] In mechanically ventilated patients, pneumonia has become one of the most difficult disease entities to manage appropriately.[2,3]

The treatment of patients with these infections requires a thorough knowledge of surgical technique, disease processes, endogenous bacterial flora and their sensitivities to various antibiotics specific to the critical care unit, and the spectra and possible toxicities of available antibiotics.[4] In addition, information on commonly recovered organisms causing nosocomial infections and their sensitivities in sputum, blood, and wounds should always be available from the hospital microbiologist. The complex issue of selecting the appropriate antimicrobial agent for the treatment of an infected critically ill patient is best resolved by a multidisciplinary team of specialists, composed of a surgeon, a physician expert in infectious disease, a microbiologist, and a pharmacist.

In this section we present the principles of antimicrobial therapy that we currently follow in our institution and discuss new pharmacodynamic concepts that are changing the dosage and administration of some antimicrobials. We also review the management of the most common surgical infections seen following trauma and in the SICU.

INFECTION

Infection vs colonization

Infection is defined as an invasion of microorganisms into tissues that normally are sterile, with subsequent initiation of the inflammatory response. This is distinguished from colonization, which is an invasion of microorganisms without signs of local or systemic inflammation. When host defense mechanisms are not sufficient, the use of antimicrobials may help to ameliorate infection. It is important to remember that, in some patients, the causative organism will be eliminated by the antimicrobials but the disease process will continue due to a toxic effect or the persistence of the systemic inflammatory response initiated by the invading microorganisms.

Microorganisms

Microorganisms often involved in surgical infections include viruses; prokaryotic organisms, such as bacteria, spirochetes, rickettsia, and chlamydiae; and eukaryotic organisms, such as fungi and parasites.[5] Most surgical infections result from host interactions with microorganisms that compromise the normal flora.

Viruses

Viruses are the smallest of all infectious agents and consist only of an inner core of RNA or DNA and a surrounding protein coat. They are obligate intracellular parasites because they lack any of the biosynthetic machinery to synthesize proteins. Their genetic materials are incorporated within that of the host cell, and it is the host cells' machinery that actually synthesizes and secretes the viral proteins. Viruses cause disease through cell lysis or alterations of cell function.

Three DNA viruses that commonly cause infection in immunocompromised surgical patients are herpes simplex virus, varicella-zoster virus, and cytomegalovirus (CMV). Pneumonia and hepatitis are common manifestations of CMV infection, and CMV has been shown to be a factor in the exacerbation of pulmonary morbidity following major trauma.[6]

Prokaryotic organisms

Prokaryotic organisms have a true cell wall but lack a distinct nucleus with a nuclear membrane. They are the smallest organisms capable of synthesizing all of the necessary proteins to sustain life independently. Bacteria are the most common prokaryotic organisms involved in surgical infections, and are classified as gram-positive or gram-negative. Gram-positive organisms have a fairly thick peptidoglycan wall and an inner plasma membrane whereas gram-negative organisms have a very thin peptidoglycan wall, an inner plasma membrane, and an outer cellular membrane. These are typical phospholipid bilayer membranes.

Many bacteria cause disease by the production of exotoxins, which are peptides that are synthesized within the cell and then released outside with a separate toxic effect. These include various streptococcal and staphylococcal toxins; tetanus toxins; a variety of toxins that lead to gas gangrene, diphtheria, and whooping cough; and a neurotoxin elaborated by Shigella that produces dysentery.

Gram-negative organisms

Endotoxins and the signs and symptoms of gram-negative sepsis

Gram-negative organisms contain a cell-associated toxic component called endotoxin, which is a lipopolysaccharide protein complex attached to the outer membrane of the gram-negative bacterial envelope that projects into the capsule, if one is present. Endotoxin consists of a lipid moiety, which is felt to be responsible for most of the toxic systemic effects of the organism; a core polysaccharide that is common to most Enterobacteriaceae; and antigen polysaccharides, which are highly variable among the gram-negative bacteria. Endotoxin has been shown in experimental animals and humans to replicate most of the signs and symptoms of gram-negative sepsis,[7] including tachycardia, tachypnea, hypotension, initiation of the complement cascade, disseminated intravascular coagulation with concomitant thrombocytopenia, the release of adrenal corticotropic hormones, and altered protein carbohydrate and lipid metabolism. Radiolabeled endotoxin injected into experimental animals has been shown to localize in the macrophages of the reticuloendothelial system, particularly in the Kupffer's cells of the liver, alveolar macrophages, and splenic macrophages. There are specific receptors on the macrophage surface for endotoxin binding and phagocytosis; once inside the cell endotoxin stimulates subsequent macrophage cytokine release. Important cytokines secreted by macrophages in this situation include interleukin (IL)-1, tumor necrosis factor, and IL-6, which

Endotoxin binding to macrophages

act to mediate the overall inflammatory response, particularly in a paracrine fashion within a given organ.[3,4,8]

Eukaryotes and fungal surgical infections

Eukaryotic organisms, which include fungi and parasites, have a true nucleus with a nuclear membrane. The most common eukaryotic organisms that produce surgical infections are fungi with low pathogenic potential, such as *Candida albicans* and *Aspergillus* sp. These organisms are likely to produce disease in patients who are granulocytopenic or have cellular immunodeficiencies. Patients receiving broad-spectrum antibiotics for an extended period are at risk of infection by these opportunistic fungi due to changes in the gut flora. Other patients at risk include those in whom a catheter has been left in place for an extended time, and patients with hyperalimentation.

Host Defenses

Table 1

Host defenses may be categorized as nonspecific or specific (Table 1). Nonspecific, or general, host defenses interfere with a microorganism's ability to cause disease. Such defenses include mechanical barriers, such as the skin and gastrointestinal tract, and various mechanisms that are stimulated by the invasion of microorganisms, such as the release of cytokines, complement, inflammatory mediators, and the process of phagocytosis itself. These host defenses are directed against all foreign antigens regardless of whether the host has been challenged previously.

Mediators of nonspecific host defenses

All host defenses are modulated by several regulatory mediators, known as cytokines. These hormone-like polypeptides are produced in response to invasion by microorganisms, and can influence the activity of multiple cells, especially lymphoid and neuroendocrine cells. Many of the symptoms associated with infectious diseases, such as fever, muscle aches, loss of appetite, and sleepiness, are due to cytokine activity.

Other mediators of the inflammatory response include histamine, kinins, and arachidonic acid metabolites. Tissue injury results in the release of histamine from mast cells, and the production of bradykinin and kallidin. These substances act directly on the vascular endothelium to increase the permeability and accumulation of cellular and protein elements of the immune system at the site of injury. Arachidonic acid is produced by a breakdown of cellular membranes and the action of phospholi-

Table 1. Classification of Host Defenses

Nonspecific	Specific
Mechanical barriers	Macrophage antigen presentation
Complement	T lymphocytes
Mediators	(cytotoxic T-cell activation)
Cytokines	B lymphocytes
Phagocytosis	(antibody production)

(From Cheadle WG. *J Royal Coll Surg [Edinb]* 1992;37:1. Reprinted with permission.)

pase A. It is then degraded by lipooxygenase to form leukotrienes, or by cyclooxygenase to form prostaglandins and thromboxanes. These eicosanoids have a variety of effects that mediate the inflammatory process. Most of the inflammatory mediators are formed quickly and locally where their effect is maximum and short-lived because of rapid metabolism.

The complement cascade

The complement cascade is a series of enzymatic cleavage reactions that are triggered by antigen-antibody complexes (classical pathway) or bacterial cell wall components (alternate pathway) and must occur in sequential fashion for efficacy. The latter pathway does not require prior exposure and, thus, represents a mechanism for immediate defense against microbial invasion. The membrane attack complex is capable of direct bacterial lysis, and activates complement anaphylatoxin components C3a and C5a to increase capillary permeability and tissue edema. Thus, complement components are capable of recruiting neutrophils by acting as chemotactants, and facilitate phagocytosis and bacterial killing by the opsonization of bacteria and the stimulation of neutrophil degranulation.[8]

Phagocytosis

The process of phagocytosis is essential to the eradication of most live invading bacteria and is carried out primarily by neutrophils and tissue macrophages.[9] It is a multiple-step process that includes adherence of the phagocytic cells to capillary endothelium; migration to the site of inflammation through chemotaxis; opsonization of the foreign material, primarily by complement or immunoglobulins; engulfment of the microbes into the cell; and, finally, microbial killing and degradation. The process is as dependent on intrinsic neutrophil function as it is on the surrounding milieu for optimal function. Disorders of phagocytosis range from low neutrophil production to defective degranulation and microbial killing and are associated with an increased risk of infection.

Specific host defenses

The specific host defenses include B and T lymphocytes, and antigen-presenting cells, such as macrophages. Foreign antigen recognition, uptake, degradation, and expression on the cell surface of the macrophage is probably the initial step in the specific immune response. Interleukin-1 is produced, and T-helper (CD4) cells bind to the foreign antigen in contiguity with the class II histocompatibility antigen HLA-DR on the macrophage cell surface. The activated CD4 cell then produces IL-2, which stimulates the maturation of B cells into plasma cells, with subsequent antibody production. Antibodies produced in this way are specific for the original foreign antigen, and memory B cells become capable of an intense secondary response to previously recognized antigen. T-suppressor (CD8) cells also may be activated by the beginning process, particularly if prostaglandin E_2 is released by macrophages. These suppressor lymphocytes probably inhibit their CD4 counterparts. Nonspecific participants, such as cytokines, inflammatory mediators, and participants involved in the process of phagocytosis itself, often are dependent on specific components as well. Phagocytosis is much more efficient for opsonized antigens and, in general, specific participants amplify the nonspecific response.

ANTIMICROBIAL THERAPY

The clinical use of antimicrobials can be classified as prophylactic when they prevent infections and therapeutic when they treat infections. The therapeutic use of antimicrobials can be categorized as empiric therapy, known pathogen therapy, or switch therapy (Fig. 1). In empiric therapy the antimicrobial is used initially to kill the most likely pathogen, in known pathogen therapy the antimicrobial is used to kill the specific microorganism known to cause the infection, and in switch therapy the antimicrobial is changed early, from a parenteral to an oral antibiotic.

Figure 1

Prophylactic Therapy

Surgical Wounds. In 1957 Miles demonstrated that there was a 4-hour window during which an antibiotic must be administered to have a protective effect against wound infection, and in 1969 Polk showed that tissue levels of an antibiotic must be two to four times greater than the minimal inhibitory concentration (MIC; the lowest antibiotic concentration at which the inhibition of bacterial growth is observed) during the course of surgery in order to be effective. This has since become standard for patients undergoing clean-contaminated operations, such as alimentary tract resection and vaginal hysterectomy, and operations in which foreign material is implanted.[10] Most surgeons feel that antibiotic coverage is necessary only during surgery—except in patients in whom foreign material is implanted—and usually indicate a safe, inexpensive, broad-spectrum first- or second-generation cephalosporin for coverage. Indeed, this has been expanded to include the treatment of patients with penetrating trauma as well. A 24-hour period of coverage with appropriate antibiotics directed against gram-negative enteric bacteria, including anaerobes, usually is sufficient.[11] It is always important

The timing of antibiotic coverage

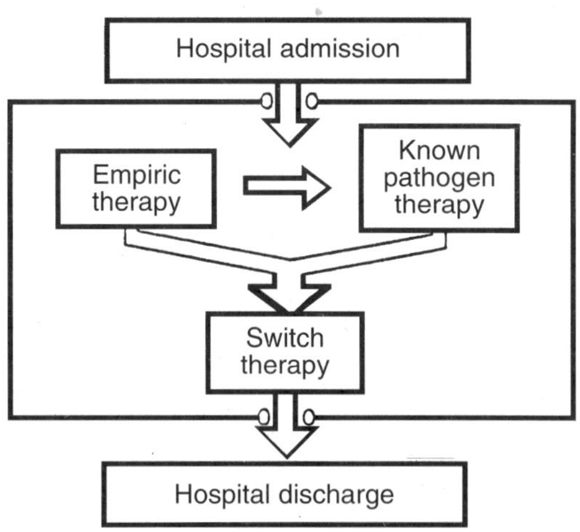

Fig. 1. The clinical use of antimicrobials in the hospital.

to achieve therapeutic levels of antimicrobials, but several recent clinical trials have documented less than adequate levels at the time of surgery.[12] Most often the antibiotic is given too early or is not redosed throughout the course of the operation. We try to administer the first dose shortly after the patient's arrival in the operating room.

Nosocomial Pneumonia. Nosocomial pneumonia is associated with the highest mortality of all nosocomial infections. One novel method of managing this problem is selective decontamination of the digestive tract (SDD), typically using a nonabsorbable antimicrobial mixture, such as a combination of nystatin, polymyxin (PMX), and gentamicin. The underlying presumption is that nosocomial pneumonia originates from the colonization of potentially pathogenic organisms in the oropharyngeal and gastrointestinal tract.[13] By eliminating these organisms, but not the indigenous flora, it may be possible to decrease the incidence of nosocomial pneumonia. Yet, three issues need to be resolved before SDD can be employed widely: Does it improve patient outcome, is there clear evidence that it does not promote the development of antibiotic resistance, and is it cost-effective? Although most studies have shown SDD to lower the incidence of nosocomial pneumonia, there is little or no evidence that it improves survival[14] and, based on the current body of evidence, we do not recommend the use of SDD at our institution.[15]

SDD not recommended for nosocomial pneumonia prophylaxis

Urinary Tract Infections. Patients with urinary catheters are at risk of sepsis originating in the urinary tract. The use of prophylactic antibiotics in this area is controversial. Based on the findings of prospective studies, we do not recommend the prophylactic use of antimicrobials in patients receiving short- or long-term urinary catheterization at our institution.

Antimicrobial prophylaxis not recommended for urinary catheter patients

Empiric Therapy

In the management of critical care infections all initial antimicrobial use is empiric. Before the initiation of antimicrobial therapy, appropriate specimens should be obtained for stains and cultures. In a significant proportion of patients cultures will be negative and the antibiotic therapy will remain empiric for its entire course. Appropriate empiric antibiotic therapy is based on reasonable educated guesses in response to the questions, what are the likely organisms causing the infection, and what are their likely susceptibility patterns?

Determining the likely pathogens

To delineate the likely pathogens, the surgeon should consider the site of infection, characteristics of the host, and results of Gram's staining of material obtained from the presumed infection site. For example, if the lung is believed to be the site of infection in a hospitalized patient on mechanical ventilation, and a Gram's stain of pulmonary secretions shows gram-negative rods, the likely etiologic pathogens would be *Pseudomonas aeruginosa* and Enterobacteriaceae.

Use of the antibiogram

Once a list of likely pathogens is obtained, the surgeon must determine their likely susceptibility. To do this, he or she should look at the history of microbial susceptibility at his or her institution. This information can be obtained from the hospital

Geographic variations in microbial susceptibility

antibiogram. It is important to recognize that there are geographic variations in the microbial susceptibility of hospital flora. For example, the susceptibility of *Escherichia coli* isolates from the institution as a whole may be 90% to a first-generation cephalosporin. However, if one analyzes *E coli* isolates taken only from the ICU, one may find that their susceptibility to the same antibiotic is only 60%. These different susceptibilities are, in part, secondary to the patterns of antimicrobial use in critically ill patients. In ICUs, antibiotic pressure favors the development of multiple-drug resistance in many bacterial species. Because of these geographic variations in susceptibility, a separate antibiogram is necessary for each critical care unit (CCU). The hospital antibiogram should report the hospital susceptibility as a whole, excluding the critical care areas. This type of susceptibility report is called a focused antibiogram. Such reports are available at our institution, and are updated every 6 months.

Using the "antibiotic failure rate" as a guide to empiric therapy

We believe that for an antibiotic to be used as empiric therapy it should have at least 80% susceptibility against the likely organisms. Based on antibiotic sensitivity, we have developed the concept of the antibiotic failure rate.[16] This is based on the resistance pattern of an antibiotic to a particular organism. For example, if tobramycin has a sensitivity of 90% against a *P aeruginosa* living in a particular CCU, the resistance pattern will be 10%. If we use tobramycin empirically to ameliorate *P aeruginosa* in this particular unit, we will fail to eliminate one out of ten infections. On the other hand, if gentamicin has a sensitivity of 80% to the same *P aeruginosa*, with a 20% resistance pattern, we will fail to eliminate one out of five infections. Table 2 lists the predicted failure rates of different antibiotics, based on their sensitivities. Antibiotics with a failure rate of one out of five infections or higher should not be used as empiric therapy.

Table 2

Monotherapy vs combination therapy

Once the surgeon has identified the best antibiotic or antibiotics to be used, he or she should decide between monotherapy and combination therapy. Monotherapy entails the coverage of one pathogen by one antibiotic, and combination therapy entails the coverage of one pathogen by two antibiotics. For example, if aztreonam and cefazolin are used in the management of nosocomial pneumonia when *P aeruginosa* is a likely pathogen, the regimen will be considered monotherapy since a single

Table 2. Determination of Antibiotic Failure Rate by Level of Resistance of a Particular Bacterial Species to an Antibiotic

Antibiotic	Bacterial Species	
	Susceptible (%)	Failure Rate
A	99	1/100
B	90	1/10
C	80	1/5
D	70	1/3

(From Ramirez.[16] Reprinted with permission.)

antibiotic is used to cover *P aeruginosa*. On the other hand, if piperacillin and tobramycin are used in the management of nosocomial pneumonia, the regimen will be considered combination therapy. Combination therapy may be beneficial by minimizing the emergence of resistant organisms and providing synergistic bactericidal activity. It is usually indicated in surgical patients when *P aeruginosa*, *Enterobacter* sp, *Acinetobacter* sp, or enterococci are considered the likely offending organisms.

Combination therapy with a β-lactam and an aminoglycoside

Combination therapy most often involves the administration of a β-lactam and an aminoglycoside antibiotic. In this way synergism is achieved because the β-lactam, acting at the level of the bacterial cell wall, enhances the penetration of the aminoglycoside, which acts at the level of protein synthesis. Combination therapy with two β-lactam antibiotics may be used in some patients to avoid the potential toxicity associated with the aminoglycosides.

Combination therapy with a β-lactam and a quinolone

A new form of combination therapy against resistant gram-negative bacteria uses a β-lactam and a quinolone antibiotic. In this regimen the β-lactam antibiotic acts at the level of the bacterial cell wall while the quinolone acts at the level of the bacterial DNA. Ongoing clinical studies will delineate the effectiveness of this form of combination therapy. In our institution, when combination therapy is indicated, we favor a regimen of a β-lactam and an aminoglycoside antibiotic.

Dosage determination

One last important consideration in the choice of initial empiric therapy is the dose of a particular antibiotic. The activity of an antibiotic is usually evaluated by the MIC. Animal models have demonstrated that the bacterial killing rate of certain antibiotics will remain maximal as long as the antibiotic level remains above the MIC for a prolonged time. Once the level of these antibiotics exceeds the MIC, further increases in their dose will not increase their activity. These agents are classified as time-dependent killing antibiotics, and include the β-lactams. A new dosing strategy is to administer the β-lactams by constant infusion to maintain the serum antibiotic concentrations above the MIC. This methodology is still under clinical investigation.

Time-dependent killing antibiotics

Animal models also have demonstrated that the bacterial killing rate of other antibiotics is maximal when a high peak concentration is reached. These agents are classified as concentration-dependent killing antibiotics, and include the aminoglycosides and quinolones. Because one would want to achieve a high ratio between the peak level of these agents and the MIC,[17] attention has been given to the possibility of administering aminoglycosides once daily. With this type of regimen there is a prolonged period during which the serum level falls below the MIC. This is associated with a decreased accumulation of the aminoglycoside in the renal cortex, and decreased renal toxicity. However, the inhibition of bacterial growth will continue due to the drugs' postantibiotic effects.

Concentration-dependent killing antibiotics

An in-hospital study

In a study we conducted at our hospital, 97% of patients with severe pneumonia who received gentamicin or tobramycin, 5 mg/kg, once daily, achieved initial peak serum levels of greater than 8 μg/mL, which is considered optimal. In contrast, patients who received conventional dosage regimens of gentamicin or tobramycin (every 8 hours) achieved suboptimal peak serum levels. All of the patients who were dosed once daily had serum trough levels below 1.5 mg/mL, whereas 20% of the patients who were dosed every 8 hours had serum trough levels in excess of 2 mg/mL. Thus, based on our experience and that of other investigators,[18-21] we have chosen to administer aminoglycosides once daily for the treatment of critically ill patients with serious gram-negative infections.

Known Pathogen Therapy

Changing to narrow-spectrum antibiotic therapy to avoid resistant organisms

Known pathogen therapy is administered to patients when the microorganism causing their infection, and its susceptibility pattern, are known. If, during empiric therapy, the patient was started on combination or broad-spectrum antibiotics, the antimicrobial spectrum is narrowed and therapy is continued with a narrow-spectrum antibiotic to avoid colonization with resistant organisms and superinfection.

Switch Therapy

Candidates for switch to oral therapy

Choice of oral agents based on pharmacokinetics and antimicrobial activity

In switch therapy there is an early replacement of the intravenous administration of antimicrobial agents with the oral dosing of antimicrobial agents which is then carried through to the completion of therapy. Switch therapy can be applied safely to patients with pulmonary, skin, soft-tissue, urinary tract, and intra-abdominal infections who have no clinical indication for intravenous therapy (eg, meningitis, endocarditis), no clinical indication of abnormal gastrointestinal drug absorption (eg, diarrhea), no fever, improving or resolved signs and symptoms related to the infection, and a normalizing white blood cell count.[22,23] The choice of oral antimicrobial agents for switch therapy should be based on the pharmacokinetics and microbiologic activity of the individual agent.

Of note, the great majority of patients do not require intravenous therapy for the completion of their antimicrobial regimen; however, it is almost always required initially in patients with serious infections, to ensure that blood levels remain above the MIC of a particular microorganism. In patients with infections localized in areas of poor antibiotic penetration, such as patients with meningitis or endocarditis, high-dose intravenous therapy is recommended for the duration of treatment.

Antimicrobial Agents

For treating patients with surgical infections, the surgeon must be familiar with the multitude of antibiotic agents currently available, as well as antifungal and antiviral agents.

Due to the predominance of gram-negative organisms seen in critically ill patients, the initial empiric regimen generally consists of a β-lactam antibiotic with or without an aminoglycoside. The prototypical β-lactam molecule has been modified repeatedly to produce the penicillin, cephalosporin, monobactam, and carbapenem classes of antibiotics. Structurally, these agents share a four-member β-lactam ring that interferes with bacterial cell wall synthesis.[24]

Penicillins

The penicillins can be classified by generation. Penicillin G is a first-generation penicillin. Penicillinase-resistant penicillins, such as nafcillin and oxacillin, which were developed to combat the penicillinase-producing *Staphylococcus aureus*, are second-generation penicillins. The first penicillin with activity against Enterobacteriaceae was ampicillin, a third-generation penicillin. The antipseudomonal penicillins are fourth-generation penicillins, and include carbenicillin, ticarcillin, mezlocillin, and piperacillin. The latest additions to the penicillin family are the fifth-generation penicillins, which are combinations of penicillins and β-lactamase inhibitors. The most commonly used antibiotics of this group are ampicillin-sulbactam, ticarcillin–clavulanic acid, and piperacillin-tazobactam. The cephalosporin antibiotics are derived from the *Cephalosporium* mold and are chemically altered to produce the varied antibiotics comprising this group.

Cephalosporins

The cephalosporins also can be classified by generation, based primarily on the increased spectrum of coverage of gram-negative organisms. First-generation cephalosporins have adequate *S aureus* (methicillin-sensitive) coverage, second-generation cephalosporins have less methicillin-sensitive coverage, and third-generation cephalosporins have the least methicillin-sensitive coverage. However, the gram-negative coverage does broaden and includes virtually all of the members of the Enterobacteriaceae family. *Pseudomonas aeruginosa* is sensitive only to ceftazidime.

Aztreonam is the only antibiotic in the group of monobactams. Its antibacterial spectrum is unique among the β-lactam antibiotics in that it is active only against gram-negative aerobes, with little or no activity against gram-positive aerobes or anaerobes.

From the group of carbapenem antibiotics, imipenem is the only one in clinical use, but this antibiotic has the widest activity of all of the β-lactam antibiotics.

Table 3

Other antibiotics commonly used in surgical patients are vancomycin, metronidazole, clindamycin, and the quinolones (Table 3).

Table 3. Commonly Used Antibiotics for Infected Patients in the Surgical Intensive Care Unit

β-Lactam Antibiotics	**Aminoglycosides**	**Quinolones**
Penicillins	Gentamicin	Ciprofloxacin
Cephalosporins	Tobramycin	Norfloxacin
Monobactams	Amikacin	Ofloxacin
Carbapenems		
β-Lactamase Production	Anti-MRSA	Antifungals
	Vancomycin	Nystatin
		Ketoconazole
		Amphotericin B

Antiendotoxin Therapy

Antibodies Against Endotoxin. Several modes of therapy have been attempted for endotoxin inhibition. In one clinical trial, polyclonal serum was shown to lower mortality from gram-negative sepsis, but the issue of potential disease transmission from multiple donors has made polyclonal antibody use unacceptable. Recombinant techniques have given rise to monoclonal antibodies (mAbs), two of which, E5 and HA-1A, have reached clinical trials.[25]

Monoclonal antibodies

E5 is a murine monoclonal immunoglobulin (Ig) M antibody. It is raised in mice immunized with *E coli* J5 that binds to an epitope on lipid. HA-1A is a human IgM mAb that binds to lipid A. It was derived from a heterohybridoma created from human spleen cells. Both mAbs have been shown to ameliorate physiologic effects in animals and the response to endotoxin as well as gram-negative bacteria. However, at a meeting of the Food and Drug Administration (FDA) in 1991, it was noted that the results of the investigations of these mAbs were not consistently reproducible, and it appeared that the bases for the clinical trials were not borne out by further preclinical studies. There has not been an experimental model in which HA-1A has consistently protected animals from an endotoxin challenge.

Trials of E5 show limited success

E5 has been tested in two placebo-controlled clinical trials. In the first, the mAb demonstrated a benefit only in patients with proved gram-negative sepsis who were not in shock. Therefore, a second trial was undertaken, involving 847 patients with suspected gram-negative sepsis who were not in shock. However, among 530 patients in whom gram-negative bacteria was documented, E5 did not improve survival.

Trials of HA-1A point to need for fundamental developments

HA-1A has been studied in a single randomized placebo-controlled trial, in which it was shown to decrease mortality in patients with gram-negative bacteremia regardless of whether they were in shock. However, several problems were noted with this study. The protective effect of HA-1A was seen only at clinical centers where there was a high placebo-related mortality and only among patients who were in shock.[26] Additionally, mortality was significantly improved only after 28 days, not after 14 days. Although benefit was originally claimed in patients who were and were not in shock, reanalysis by the FDA demonstrated no benefit in patients who were not in shock. The investigators came to the conclusion that only patients who had gram-negative bacteremia and were in shock might benefit from HA-1A. Another problem with this trial was that patients with inadequate antimicrobial chemotherapy were not excluded, yet had a higher mortality.

An accurate determination of efficacy is especially important for HA-1A because the drug is likely to benefit only a small subset of patients at an extremely high cost. Estimates are $3,500 per dose in Europe and more than $4,000 per dose in the United States of America. A second trial of this mAb had to be stopped because of too many deaths in the HA-1A arm. At this point HA-1A will have to undergo additional fundamental development before further clinical study. Patients who should be entered into future trials are those with presumed gram-negative bacteremia and septic shock.[27]

Polymyxin B

Adsorption of Endotoxin. Polymyxin B is a cyclic cationic polypeptide antibiotic that inactivates endotoxin. When administered intravenously to dogs it was shown to neutralize the hemodynamic effects on blood pressure and systemic vascular resistance caused by gram-negative endotoxin. However, its intravenous use is limited by its nephrotoxicity. To avoid this problem, PMX-B has been bound covalently to an insoluble polystyrene fiber (PMX-F) and since been used in experiments as a filter ex vivo during extracorporeal circulation in conjunction with systemic antibiotics. In theory, PMX-F binds with endotoxin and alters its biologic activity through stereochemical changes. The systemic side effects of intravenous PMX-B are avoided because the PMX-F does not release PMX-B into the bloodstream. This method, combined with antibiotics and nonspecific immune stimulation, was found to improve survival in dogs and rats subjected to lethal doses of intravenous gram-negative endotoxin or live *E coli*.[28] More recent work from a multicenter study in Japan has shown increased survival in patients undergoing endotoxin filtration by venovenous dialysis.[29]

Monophosphoryl lipid A

Lipid A Analogues. Monophosphoryl lipid (MPL) A, an analogue of lipid A that lacks one side chain, has been used prophylactically in a variety of animal models, rendering animals more resistant to gram-negative and gram-positive bacteria as well as to endotoxin challenge. In addition, animals immunized with liposomes containing MPL have shown increased resistance to subsequent challenge in bacteria and endotoxin.[30] Although these animals developed antibodies to lipid A, titers did not correlate with survival or other measures of immune function, such as macrophage activation. Clinical trials are under way in which MPL A is being given to patients with a high probability of developing sepsis or septic shock. Obviously, the selection of such patients is difficult, and trying to prove efficacy in a randomized trial will require a tremendous number of participants.

COMMON SURGICAL INFECTIONS

Urinary tract infections, pneumonia, peritonitis, and catheter-related infections comprise the vast majority of infections in critical care patients. In our own series of severely injured patients, pneumonia was the most common serious infection, followed by peritonitis and intra-abdominal abscess formation. The most common pathogens isolated in the SICU are listed in Table 4 (see page 34).

Table 4

Urinary Tract Infections

Causes and control of urinary tract infections

Although infection of the urinary tract is the most common nosocomial infection, it is fairly easy to control if obstruction is not present. In surgical patients, urinary tract infections are related directly to the length of time a catheter is left in the bladder; their incidence increases markedly after 1 week of bladder catheterization. *Escherichia coli* and other gram-negative organisms are the usual causative agents, and antibiotics that cover these pathogens should be used for empiric therapy.

Nosocomial Pneumonia

Approximately 300,000 cases of nosocomial pneumonia occur annually in the United States of America, with an associated mortality of 20% to 50%. Pneumonia is the leading cause of death from nosocomial infection. It effects surgical patients as an isolated infection and a concomitant infection, particularly with infections arising from within the abdomen. Nosocomial pneumonias are defined as pneumonias that occur from 48 to 72 hours after hospital admission. This definition has important implications for antibiotic therapy because the likely pathogens and their respective sensitivities differ from those for community-acquired pneumonias.[31] Patients in intensive care and postsurgical recovery units are at the greatest risk of contracting nosocomial pneumonia, primarily as a result of the subclinical aspiration of bacteria colonizing the upper airways. Intubation, surgical stress, underlying chronic pulmonary diseases, and exposure to gram-negative hospital flora are risk factors for the development of nosocomial pneumonia. The use of histamine$_2$ antagonists and antacids for the prevention of stress ulcers has been identified as another potential risk factor, but a study comparing the efficacy of sucralfate with these agents in stress ulcer patients found an increased incidence of pneumonia among the sucralfate-treated subjects, although this was not clinically significant.[32]

The definition of nosocomial pneumonias

Gram-negative bacillary pathogens are the predominant etiologic agents causing nosocomial pneumonia. *Pseudomonas aeruginosa* and Enterobacteriaceae (eg, *E coli*, *Klebsiella* sp, *Enterobacter* sp, and *Proteus* sp) account for more than 60% of all cases. In addition, *S aureus* accounts for approximately 10% to 15% of cases. Of these, approximately 20% to 30% will be resistant to methicillin, necessitating expensive and potentially toxic treatment with vancomycin.[33]

Causes of nosocomial pneumonia

It is often difficult to diagnose nosocomial pneumonia because of preexisting confounding factors. Risk factors in the trauma patient include severe head injury, emergent intubation, and shock; such patients have been shown to benefit by early tracheostomy.[34] Clinical symptoms, such as fever, cough, produc-

Difficulties in diagnosis

Table 4. Most Common Bacterial Pathogens Isolated From the University of Louisville Hospital Surgical Intensive Care Unit

Pathogen	Incidence
Staphylococcus aureus	24%
Enterobacter sp	18%
Pseudomonas sp	11%
Staphylococcus epidermidis	9%
Escherichia coli	7%
Acinetobacter sp	6%
Klebsiella sp	5%

tive sputum, and chest pain, may not be present in the hospitalized patient. Most of these critically ill patients have moderate leukocytosis and an underlying infiltrate, visible on chest x-ray, due to fluid resuscitation, pulmonary contusion, or progressive atelectasis. Additionally, the isolation of potentially pathogenic bacteria from cultures of the respiratory tract does not necessarily confirm the presence of pneumonia, as colonization may occur in the absence of infection. Abrupt changes in clinical status, such as fever, oxygenation parameters, and sputum production in combination with a new or changing infiltrate on chest x-ray lead to the diagnosis of nosocomial pneumonia.

Control of nosocomial pneumonia

Initial treatment is supportive, with increased inspired oxygen, positive end-expiratory pressure, tracheal suction, percussion, bronchoscopy, and frequent placement of the patient in the upright position, preferably in a chair. Early, empiric antibiotic treatment with broad-spectrum therapy sufficient to cover gram-negative and gram-positive organisms is instituted prior to obtaining final culture results regardless of the type of bacteria noted on Gram's stain. Conventional therapy has evolved to include the administration of penicillins or cephalosporins, each in combination with an aminoglycoside. More recently, single-agent antibiotic therapy with the broad-spectrum β-lactam antibiotics has been used clinically.[35] Empiric monotherapy usually consists of a penicillin combined with a β-lactamase inhibitor (eg, ticarcillin–clavulanic acid, piperacillin-tazobactam); a carbapenem with a renal dehydropeptidase inhibitor (eg, imipenem-cilastatin); a cephalosporin (eg, cefoxitin, ceftazidime); or a monobactam (eg, aztreonam). When aztreonam is used as empiric therapy for nosocomial pneumonia it should be combined with cefazolin or vancomycin.

Intra-Abdominal Infections

Primary bacterial peritonitis

Secondary bacterial peritonitis

Tertiary bacterial peritonitis

Peritonitis can be classified as primary, secondary, or tertiary. Primary peritonitis (spontaneous bacterial peritonitis) used to be a disease of historical interest that disappeared with the advent of the antibiotic era. It has resurfaced with the common use of paracentesis in patients with liver disease and ascites, and with the advent of continuous ambulatory peritoneal dialysis in patients with renal failure. Secondary bacterial peritonitis may be caused by inflammation of the hollow viscera, perforated peptic ulcer, acute cholecystitis, diverticulitis, appendicitis, and perforation of the small intestine. With the exception of diverticular disease, these disorders require surgery for definitive treatment if they have not produced an abscess or obstruction. Secondary bacterial peritonitis also may arise from complications of elective surgery, requiring reoperation or radiologic-guided drainage for definitive treatment. Tertiary bacterial peritonitis is peritonitis that recurs after an operation for peritonitis, such as surgery for pancreatic abscess or hollow viscus perforation. As such, it is often associated with the septic state and multiple organ failure.

In general, antibiotic therapy for peritonitis consists of gentamicin and clindamycin. However, because of the toxicity

Treatment

associated with these two antibiotics, a number of clinical and experimental studies have used broad-spectrum β-lactam antibiotics with equally good results. Unfortunately, these clinical studies have been difficult to interpret because of an inability to compare patients and sites of infection. This was formally recognized by the Surgical Infection Society, which set up a committee to draft appropriate criteria for the proper conduct of clinical trials.[36] Dellinger showed that mortality in patients with peritonitis was closely correlated with the acute physiology score but not with the site of inflammation, except in cases of appendicitis. Evidence has shown that a broad-spectrum cephalosporin is as efficacious as the combination of clindamycin and an aminoglycoside, or imipenem/cilastatin.[37] Future trials of antibiotic regimens in the treatment of patients with peritonitis will need to be properly stratified as outlined by site of infection as well as acute physiology score.

Catheter-Related Infections

Table 5

Although the overall risk of catheter-related infections is very low, these infections are fairly common because of the tremendous number of catheters currently in use. Table 5 lists several risk factors for catheter-related infections; other risks include total parenteral nutrition, immunosuppression, and remote infections.[38] A documented catheter-related infection requires replacement of the catheter at a different site, often the administration of intravenous antibiotics, and an extended stay in the ICU or hospital. The most commonly recovered organisms in catheter-related infections are *S epidermidis*, *S aureus* and, occasionally, yeast. Most often these are caused by the migration of microbes from the skin down the catheter tract. Indeed, all catheters are associated with a surrounding fibrin-laden film and clot that often becomes the site of colonization and subsequent infection. However, contamination through the solution infused into the catheter or hematogenous spread from remote sites may occur. Indeed, piggyback ports have been developed to reduce the risk of infection during catheter tubing changes.

Causes of catheter-related infection

The incidence of infection is actually lower with central lines placed through the subclavian vein than with lines placed through the internal jugular vein, although the risk of pneumothorax and life-threatening venous bleeding from vein laceration is higher. The rate of infection varies inversely with the length of the catheter tubing from underneath the skin to the synthetic polyester cuff in permanent catheters. Therefore, it is important to place the cuff as far as possible from the dermal exit site. Obviously, sources in the head and neck are preferable to those in the groin because of the increased concentrations of skin flora in this area. However, if no upper access exists, groin catheters can be used for prolonged periods. In such cases, a partially occlusive dressing is best; a simple povidone-iodine–moistened gauze changed once or twice daily is associated with the lowest risk of catheter infection.

Catheter placement

Problems with plastic dressings

Transparent plastic dressings have become popular over the last few years, but studies have shown that they carry an increased risk of infection, as organisms can multiply in this moist environment. If such dressings are to be used, they need to be changed every 48 hours. Similarly, multiple-lumen catheters have become popular because of the need for multiple access ports in severely ill patients. However, these catheters are associated with a greater risk of infection than are single-lumen catheters. In reality, multiple-lumen ports are used almost universally for in-hospital care, but often there is a choice between a double-lumen externally placed permanent catheter and a single-lumen externally placed permanent catheter, and subcutaneously placed permanent catheters are virtually always single-lumen. In immunodeficient patients temporary catheters are preferred because of their relative ease of change. The rate of infection is so high in these patients that frequent changes are required, and there is less wound morbidity associated with temporary catheters.

Single- vs multiple-lumen catheters

Prophylactic antibiotics should be administered perioperatively when permanent intravascular catheters are being inserted, but are not necessary for usual triple-lumen central lines.[38] Reinsertion of a catheter over a guide wire is known to increase the risk of infection to the bloodstream.[39] Tubing from the source bag to the port should be replaced every 48 to 72 hours to

Table 5. Risk Factors for Catheter Infection and Their Modification

Factors Affecting Infection	Risk Modification Techniques
Duration of catheterization	Remove as soon as indicated
Site of insertion	Use peripheral access when possible Attempt subclavian insertion first
Concurrent infection	Treat concurrent infection Avoid use of a central catheter if possible Monitor carefully
Technique of insertion	Puncture skin at single site Use antibacterial skin preparation Use sterile technique Avoid catheter manipulation
Catheter care	Perform 48-hour skin decontamination and dressing change Avoid plastic dressings Avoid in-line tubing manipulation
Type of catheter	Use single-lumen catheter when possible Use steel needles when possible Consider antibacterial cuff catheters

maximally reduce the risk of contamination from this source.[38]

Catheter introducers and associated infection

When pulmonary artery catheters are used in the ICU, the introducer is large and associated with a marked increase in risk of infection and air embolism. Hence, as soon as the pulmonary artery catheter is removed, one should consider converting these introducers to a smaller, triple-lumen catheter. There is a tendency to leave these introducers in for a few days because of an anticipated need for replacement of the pulmonary artery catheter, or even neglect them as the patient improves. We make a special effort to remove the introducers or convert them to triple-lumen catheters within 24 hours of pulmonary artery catheter removal.

Diagnosing catheter-related infections

Most often a diagnosis of catheter-related infection is based on culture of the blood and the removed catheter.[40] A semiquantitative technique is used whereby the catheter is rolled in agar, and if 15 or more colonies grow, primary catheter-related infection is diagnosed. Fever, erythema, purulent drainage, and the absence of any other source of infection may lead one to suspect the catheter; in such cases the catheter should be removed. However, fever occurs more commonly in the setting of remote infection. This raises the question of whether the catheter is contributing to the infection. If other causes have been ruled out or are being remedied at that time, persistent fever and/or leukocytosis occurs, and there is no local evidence of infection, it is reasonable to change the catheter over a guide wire and culture it. If the catheter is infected the replacement catheter should be removed as well, and a new site chosen. When a positive blood culture shows the same organisms as those recovered from the catheter tip, catheter-related bacteremia has probably occurred; this should be managed with intravenous antibiotics. Vancomycin is the drug of choice for empiric therapy until final sensitivities are reported, as staphylococci are the most common cause of catheter-related infections, and most *S epidermidis* bacteria and approximately 25% to 33% of *S aureus* bacteria are resistant to methicillin. If the organisms are not resistant to methicillin, vancomycin can be switched to nafcillin to complete a 5-day course of antibiotic therapy.

Antibiotic-catheter bonding

The bonding of antibiotics to catheters has been attempted for many years. Originally silver was used successfully to achieve the antibiotic effect. More recently, silver sulfadiazine and chlorhexadine have been bonded to catheters, and their effectiveness has been demonstrated in small series. Currently we are conducting a prospective study of the use of these agents in our ICU. Catheters that are placed percutaneously into the antecubital vein and then threaded into the superior vena cava have become popular and seem to carry a lower risk of infection. If arm access is available, these catheters will probably become a first option as they also lessen some of the risks associated with central catheter placement.

CONCLUSION

Steps in proper patient management

Infection continues to confront critical care patients, and the surgeon must be ready to manage a wide variety of pathogens.

Proper patient management, including antiseptic preoperative cleansing, minimal hospital preoperative stay, bowel preparation, aseptic technique, prophylactic antibiotic administration when indicated, and vigorous postoperative care should limit the incidence of surgical wound infections. Proper knowledge of the normal flora coupled with that of the typical pathogens that affect given sites, and their sensitivities, are important for proper empiric antibiotic selection in patients who develop infections postoperatively and patients who present to the surgical service with infection. Changes in antibiotic therapy are indicated when resistant organisms are subsequently cultured, particularly if there is a lack of clinical improvement. The duration of intravenous antibiotic therapy is variable, but should continue until clinical signs and symptoms of infection are lessened or resolved. Normalization of an elevated white blood cell count is often used as a criterion for the cessation of antibiotic therapy, particularly in patients with peritonitis. The rational use of antibiotics will help the surgeon treat infected patients efficiently, with a minimal emergence of resistant bacterial strains and toxicity.[41] In the future, newer forms of therapy directed at blocking endotoxin and mediators of the inflammatory reaction may play a role in the treatment of critically ill patients with infectious diseases.

Antibiotic therapy

References

1. Howard RJ, Simmons RL (eds). *Surgical Infectious Diseases*, ed 2. Norwalk, Ct, Appleton & Lange, 1988.
2. Clowes GA (ed). *Trauma, Sepsis, and Shock: The Physiological Basis of Therapy*. New York, NY, Marcel Dekker, Inc, 1988.
3. Baue AE, in Faist E, et al (eds). *Host Defense Dysfunction in Trauma, Shock and Sepsis*. Berlin, Germany, Springer-Verlag, 1993, pp 3-14.
4. Meakins JL (ed). *Surgical Infections: Diagnosis and Treatment*, ed 1. New York, NY, Scientific American, Inc, 1994.
5. Joklik WK, et al (eds). *Zinsser Microbiology*, Norwalk, Ct, Appleton & Lange, 1988.
6. Curtsinger LJ, et al. *Am J Surg* 1989;158:606-611.
7. Michie HR, et al. *N Engl J Med* 1988;318:1481-1486.
8. Fry DE (ed). *Multiple System Organ Failure*. St Louis, Mo, Mosby-Year Book, Inc, 1992.
9. Bryant RE, in Root R, et al (eds). *Contemporary Issues in Infectious Diseases: New Surgical and Medical Approaches*, vol 5. New York, NY, Churchill Livingstone Inc, 1987.
10. Polk HC Jr, Lopez-Mayor JF. *Surgery* 1969;66:97-103.
11. Fabian TC, et al. *Surgery* 1992;112:788-795.
12. Galandiuk S, et al. *Surg Gynecol Obstet* 1989;169:219-222.
13. Fink MP. *Crit Care Med* 1992;20:559-562.
14. Selective Decontamination of the Digestive Tract Trialists' Collaborative Group. *Br Med J* 1993;307:525-532.
15. Hammond JMJ, et al. *Crit Care Med* 1994;22:33-39.
16. Ramirez J. *J Chemother* 1994;6:47-50.
17. Moore R, et al. *J Infect Dis* 1987;155:93-99.
18. Fan ST, et al. *J Antimicrob Chemother* 1988;22:69-74.
19. Hollender LF, et al. *J Antimicrob Chemother* 1989;23:773-783.
20. TerBraak EW, et al. *Am J Med* 1990;89:58-66.
21. Maller R, et al. *J Antimicrob Chemother* 1988;22:75-79.
22. Ramirez J, et al. *Pharm Ther* 1993;18:267-273.
23. Ramirez J. *Clinician* 1993;11:38-40.
24. Donowitz GR, Mandell GL. *N Engl J Med* 1988;318:419-426.

25. Bone RC. *JAMA* 1991;266:1686-1691.
26. Warren HS, et al. *N Engl J Med* 1992;326:1153-1157.
27. Bone RC, et al. *Chest* 1992;101:1644-1655.
28. Cheadle WG, et al. *Surgery* 1991;110:785-792.
29. Kodama M, *Intensive Care Med* 1994;20(suppl 1):S153.
30. Holaday J, et al. *Intensive Care Med* 1994;20(suppl 1):S145.
31. Garner JS, et al. *Am J Infect Control* 1988;16:128-140.
32. Cioffi WG, et al. *J Trauma* 1994;36:541-547.
33. Brumfitt W, Hamilton-Miller J. *N Engl J Med* 1989;320:1188-1196.
34. Rodriguez JL, et al. *J Trauma* 1991;31:907-914.
35. Naziri W, et al. *Ann Surg* 1994;219:632-642.
36. Nystrom PO, et al. *World J Surg* 1990;14:148-158.
37. Solomkin JS, et al. *Ann Surg* 1990;212:581-591.
38. Garrison RN, Wilson MA. *Surg Clin North Am* 1994;74:557-570.
39. Cobb DK, et al. *N Engl J Med* 1992;327:1062-1068.
40. Hagley MT, et al. *Crit Care Med* 1992;20:1426-1430.
41. Hadjiminas D, et al. *Am J Surg* 1994;168:288-290.

III Cytokine Regulation of the Host Response to Sepsis

Stephen F. Lowry, MD
Steven E. Calvano, PhD

BRIEF CONTENTS

INTRODUCTION

The management of patients with severe infection and septic shock has been an area of intense scientific and clinical investigation. Such investigation has focused attention on the earlier identification and appropriate classification of infected individuals and provided greater insight into the pathophysiology and therapeutic strategies specific to severe sepsis and septic shock. Many studies have emphasized a number of significant biologic issues referable to the dysregulation of homeostasis during severe infection. In this section we profile what is currently understood of the cytokine mediator system.

Mechanisms of defense

The human body defends itself against infection with physical barriers, circulating and tissue-fixed phagocytic cells, cytotoxic T lymphocytes, and soluble circulating molecules that orchestrate and maintain immune function. Some defense mechanisms are present prior to infectious challenge and are not enhanced by single or repeated exposure to foreign molecules. This describes a phenomenon known as *innate* or *natural* immunity. Alternatively, some components of the immune response are induced or amplified by antigen exposure. This is referred to as *specific* or *acquired* immunity, as it is specific to the challenging antigen and also exhibits the capacity to increase the magnitude of the body's immune response with each succeeding exposure to that antigen.

Innate immunity

Specific immunity

Secretory products of the natural immune system serve to modify and direct its phagocytic cells as well as lymphocytes of the specific immune system to sites of antigen exposure. Here cognate and noncognate interactions occur among cells of the two systems. The hallmark of the specific immune system is its capacity to recall prior encounters with foreign antigens which, when not otherwise compromised by disease, permits increasingly enhanced defensive activity.

The orchestration of the interactions between the natural and specific immune systems requires a mechanism for regulating the magnitude and duration of their individual and complimentary

Cytokines

functions. The effector phases of both natural and specific immunity are directed, to a large extent, by proteins now commonly known as *cytokines*. These proteins are produced predominantly by mononuclear phagocytes during natural immune responses, often in direct response to microbe phagocytosis. They also may be secreted by T cells stimulated by antigen presentation, resulting in the initiation of a specific immune response. Several cytokines secreted by stimulated T lymphocytes serve to regulate the activation and expansion of lymphocyte subpopulations while other T-cell–derived cytokines direct the activity of other inflammatory cells.

CYTOKINE PROPERTIES

The cytokines are polypeptides or glycoproteins of relatively low molecular weight—generally ≤25 to 30 kD in their monomeric form, although some exert their biologic activity in their higher–molecular weight oligomeric forms. At present it appears that the production and secretion of most cytokines is of limited duration and that basal (constitutive) production is usually absent or occurs at very low levels. Further, most cytokines are not stored as preformed molecules; hence, their production requires new gene transcription and translation. The transcription of many cytokine genes generally results in an unstable messenger RNA (mRNA), providing a potential mechanism for the tight regulation of their appearance.

Cytokine activities

All cytokines exert their action by binding to specific cell surface receptors (K_d usually 10^{-9} to 10^{-12} M). In contrast to the activity of many other peptide hormones, the activity of cytokines is generally exerted over a short radius by way of binding to the cell of its origin (autocrine influence) or a neighboring target cell (paracrine influence). Some cytokines exert an influence on distal target cells (endocrine influence), although in most cases the detection of such proteins in the circulation more likely reflects excessive activity of these mediators at the tissue level.

Tables 1 and 2

Once they are bound to the target cells, the cytokines exert their postreceptor actions through second messenger systems, usually resulting in an altered pattern of gene expression. Most cellular responses to cytokines require new mRNA transcription and are relatively slow. Many of these include some component of altered cell proliferation, differentiation, or differentiated function. Hence, many cytokine species also serve as growth factors for the regulation of cell division, and most exert some influence upon hematopoietic cells. Additionally, cytokines may influence the production as well as the action of other cytokines, thus permitting an additional degree of regulation for the attenuation or amplification of their influences. Tables 1 and 2 (see pages 46 and 47) illustrate the diversity of individual cytokine activities and the number of functional properties shared by these mediators. In the discussion that follows we catalogue the cytokines that have been subjected to sufficient study to depict documented in vitro and purported in vivo immune functions.

Table 1. In Vitro Natural and Acquired Immune Cytokine* Functions

Cytokine	Cell Source	Cell Target	Primary Effects Target	Receptor MW (kD)
TNF	Mononuclear phagocytes T cells	Neutrophils Endothelial cells T and B cells	Activation (inflammation) Activation (inflammation, coagulation) Costimulator	55, 75
LT	T cells	Neutrophils Endothelial cells	Activation Activation	55, 75
IL-1α IL-1β	Mononuclear phagocytes	T and B cells Endothelial cells	Costimulator Activation (inflammation, coagulation)	60, 80 60, 80
IL-2	T_H1 cells	T cells NK cells B cells	Growth, cytokine production Growth, activation Growth, antibody synthesis	50, 64, 75
IL-4	T_H2 cells	T cells B cells	Growth Activation and growth, isotype switching to IgE	120
IL-5	T_H2 cells	Eosinophils B cells	Activation Growth and activation	60, 130
IL-6	Mononuclear phagocytes Endothelial cells T cells	T and B cells Mature B cells Hepatocytes	Costimulator Growth	80+ (gp/30)
IL-8 (Chemokines)	Mononuclear phagocytes Endothelial cells Fibroblasts T cells Platelets	Leukocytes	Leukocyte activation and chemotaxis	59, 67
IL-10	TH2 cells B cells	NK and T cells T cells Mononuclear phagocytes	Inhibits IFN-γ production Inhibits TNF production	
IL-12	Mononuclear macrophages B cells	T and NK cells	Activation	
Type I IFNs-α Type I IFNs-β	Mononuclear phagocytes, other (α), fibroblasts, other (β)	Diverse NK cells	Antiviral, antiproliferative, increased class I MHC expression Activation	α, 95–110 β, 95–110
IFN-γ	T_H2 cells NK cells	Mononuclear phagocytes Endothelial cells NK cells All	Activation	90, 95
TGF-β	T cells Mononuclear phagocytes	T cells Mononuclear phagocytes	Inhibit activation and proliferation Inhibit activation	

*Includes those cytokines for which sufficient data currently exist. (From Lowry et al. *Arch Surg* 1993;128:1235-1241. Reprinted with permission.)

CYTOKINES PRODUCED PREDOMINANTLY BY MONONUCLEAR PHAGOCYTES

Tumor Necrosis Factor

Figure 1

Tumor necrosis factor (TNF) is the most proximal cytokine mediator of the natural immune response to bacterial lipopolysaccharide (Fig. 1; see page 48).[1,2] Although several cells (eg, activated T cells, natural killer [NK] cells, mast cells) are capable of producing this potent mediator, those of mononuclear phagocyte lineage appear to be the principal source of TNF production. Tumor necrosis factor is polymorphic and can exert its activity as a transmembrane, cell-associated species and as a secreted species. It binds to either of two specific cell receptors (Table 1) with relatively low avidity and may exhibit differing characteristics at varying concentrations. At lower concentrations (10^{-9} M) it activates inflammatory neutrophils and monocytes to affect microbial killing, the stimulation of T- and B-cell function, and the expression of class I major histocompatibility complex (MHC) molecules. Tumor necrosis factor further stimulates the production of other proinflammatory cytokines (eg, interleukin [IL]-1) and specialized cytokines (eg, IL-6, IL-8) and enhances endothelial cell adhesiveness for leukocytes, thereby contributing to the recruitment of these activated cells to sites of inflammation and infection. These characteristics underscore the significant role of TNF in the process of host containment and the eradication of microbes. Likewise, these functions may serve to recognize and contain malignant cells through direct tumor lysis as well as by inducing thrombosis of tumor neovascularity.

Host containment and microbe eradication by TNF

When present at tissue sites or in excessive amounts in the circulation, TNF does promote some beneficial responses, such as increased core temperature and hepatic acute phase protein production. However, increased quantities of TNF also may be associated with a number of adverse systemic events, such as a condition of hemodynamic collapse attributable to several

Adverse systemic effects of TNF

Table 2. In Vivo Responses Potentially Attributable to Individual Cytokines*

	TNF	LT	IL-1	IL-2	IL-4	IL-5	IL-6	IL-8	IL-10	IFN
Induction of fever	Y		Y	Y						Y
Induction of acute phase protein	Y		Y				Y			Y
Induction of septic shock	Y			Y			Y		N	Y
Induction of cachexia	Y	Y		Y	?					Y

*Several cytokines with ill-defined functions in vivo are not included here.
Y = Established activity, N = no evidence of activity, ? = variably reported activities.
(From Lowry et al. *Arch Surg* 1993;128:1235-1241. Reprinted with permission.)

influences, including reduced vascular smooth muscle tone, reduced myocardial contractility, and activation of the coagulation cascade with associated intravascular thrombosis. The essential nature of TNF in systemic host deterioration from severe infection has been documented by the protective influence of anti-TNF antibodies (or free TNF receptor species).

Interleukin-1

Derivation of IL-1

Interleukin-1 shares many functions with TNF that are directed toward natural immunity and inflammatory responses.[3] Although IL-1 may be produced from lipopolysaccharide-activated mononuclear phagocytes or by TNF stimulation, it also arises from epithelial and endothelial cells. Cognate interactions between mononuclear phagocyte antigen-presenting cells and antigen-specific CD4$^+$ T cells are also efficient stimuli of IL-1 production. Two species of bioactive IL-1 are produced (α and β), although these distinct gene products share only limited amino acid sequence homology. Both IL-1 precursor species are proteolytically cleaved by an enzyme that may serve as a target for their regulation.

IL-1α

Interleukin-1α may be active in a higher molecular weight (33-kD) form or as the mature 17-kD protein. It also may exert biologic activity through a membrane-associated species.

IL-1β

By contrast, IL-1β is active only in the more mature 17-kD form. A mechanism for IL-1 secretion is not evident from the structure of the native proteins; hence, the presence of circulating forms of IL-1 in vivo may be more indicative of severe cell injury or lysis than

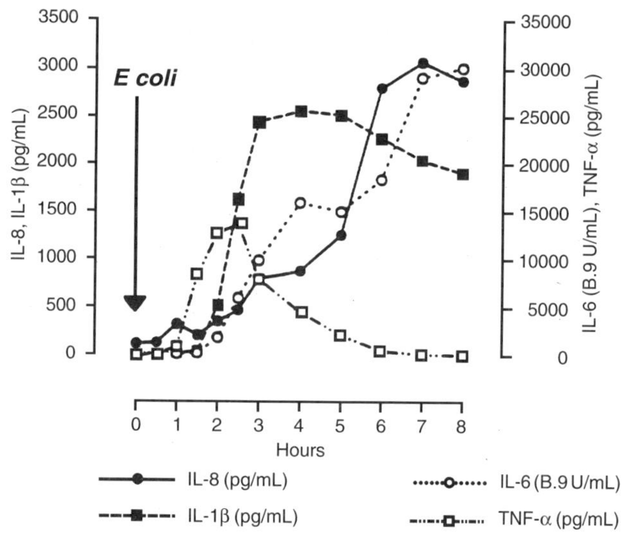

Fig. 1. Circulating cytokine levels in states of septic shock. Blood samples were obtained every 30 to 60 minutes from baboons that had received a lethal dose of live *Escherichia coli*. Mean cytokine levels for each time point are shown for TNF-α (❑), IL-1β (■), IL-6 (○), and IL-8 (●) and were determined by enzyme-linked immunosorbent assay (for TNF-α, IL-1β, and IL-8) and B.9 hybridoma proliferation assay (for IL-6).

of endogenous secretion. Nevertheless, both IL-1 species bind to either of two cell surface receptors. The mechanisms for postreceptor IL-1 activation remain controversial and several potential biochemical pathways, including that resulting in prostaglandin synthesis, may be activated.

Stimulation of cytokine mediators

A proliferation of $CD4^+$ T and B cells is observed at lower levels of IL-1 activity. The two IL-1 species also stimulate the production of other cytokine mediators, including IL-2, IL-6, and IL-8, and are inherently pyrogenic and promote components of the acute phase reaction. These cytokines do not increase the expression of class I MHC molecules nor do they exert antitumor effects directly or elicit severe tissue injury and systemic hemodynamic collapse.

Studies of an IL-1 receptor antagonist

Investigators have identified an additional member of the IL-1 family that shares some structural homology with IL-1α and IL-1β.[4] Although this species binds to the same receptors as IL-1α and IL-1β, it does not exert an agonist influence. Preclinical data suggest that this so-called IL-1 receptor antagonist (IL-1ra) may, at sufficiently high doses, prevent some sequelae of severe endotoxemia or sepsis.

Interleukin-6

Interleukin-6 is also produced by mononuclear phagocytes and other cell types in response to IL-1 and TNF.[5] However, unlike most other cytokine species, IL-6 is more readily detected systemically and, thus, serves more of a classic endocrine function. In this capacity IL-6 regulates several distinct components of the hepatic acute phase response and promotes B-cell differentiation and the costimulation of T cells. The direct influences of IL-6 on the adverse host response to severe infection remain unclear. It appears that the activation of an additional cell surface receptor complex (gp130) is necessary for the complete induction of cellular responses to this cytokine. Prior activation by TNF, the IL-1s, or any combination thereof, is contributory to the full expression of IL-6 activity.

Interleukin-8

Interleukin-8 is derived from activated mononuclear phagocytes and T cells as well as platelets.[6] It is the best-characterized member of a family of so-called chemokinetic mediators and has been shown to be chemotactic and activating for neutrophils. Interleukin-8, like IL-6, exhibits no inherent toxicity when administered exogenously.

Interleukin-10

IL-10: An inhibitory cytokine

Interleukin-10 is a 35- to 40-kD cytokine secreted by mononuclear phagocytes and a subset of T-helper cells.[7,8] Originally it was called *cytokine synthesis inhibitory factor* because of its ability to inhibit the monocyte/macrophage production of most proinflammatory cytokines, including TNF, IL-1, IL-6, and IL-8. Interleukin-10 also markedly attenuates T-cell interferon (IFN)-γ and IL-2 synthesis/secretion. These IL-10–induced decreases in levels of IFN-γ are associated with the downregulation of monocyte/

macrophage class II MHC molecules and suboptimal antigen-presenting functions. Interleukin-10 also may cause the upregulation of IL-1ra, further contributing to the inhibition of proinflammatory cytokine responses.

Interleukin-12

Originally IL-12 was identified as a 70-kD glycoprotein present in the culture supernatant of a human B lymphoblastoid cell line.[9,10] Subsequent work has shown that mononuclear phagocytes are a major source of this cytokine. When added to cultures of normal human mononuclear cells, IL-12 increases T-cell IFN-γ production, enhances NK cell cytotoxicity, and markedly increases T-cell proliferation. Because of its enhancing effects on NK cells, IL-12 was originally called *NK cell stimulating factor.*

CYTOKINES PRODUCED PREDOMINANTLY BY LYMPHOCYTES

Immune Interferon-γ

Interferon-γ is produced by $CD4^+$ and $CD8^+$ T cells in response to antigen activation and IL-2.[11] It binds to a different cell receptor than does IFN-α or IFN-β and varies functionally from those cytokines in several important respects, including a direct influence upon mononuclear phagocyte activation. Interferon-γ induces the synthesis of enzymes necessary for the respiratory burst and, hence, is also a macrophage-activating factor. Additionally, IFN-γ increases class II MHC expression and promotes the differentiation of T and B cells and the activation of NK cells.

Functions of IFN-γ

Interleukin-2

Interleukin-2 is also produced by $CD4^+$ and $CD8^+$ T cells.[12] Known principally as a cytokine responsible for promoting T-cell growth, IL-2 serves this function by both autocrine and paracrine actions. The quantity of IL-2 produced by the $CD4^+$ cells defines the magnitude of antigen-induced immune responses. Interleukin-2 also stimulates NK cell growth and function, resulting in the generation of so-called lymphokine-activated killer cells. This property has been adapted widely to the ex vivo and in vivo adoptive immunotherapy of certain malignancies. Interleukin-2 binds in a complex manner to three cell surface receptors—α, β, and γ—although growth is maximal when IL-2 cross-links all three receptors. Chronic or excessive T-cell stimulation leads to a shedding of IL-2 receptors, which has led to its use as a marker (such as that recently proposed for TNF receptors) of excessive antigen stimulation.

Stimulation of NK cell growth by IL-2

Interleukin-4

Interleukin-4 is produced by $CD4^+$ T lymphocytes yet does not share the variety of functions ascribed to the murine species. Interleukin-4 also may induce the endothelial cell binding of monocytes and lymphocytes. Additionally, recent data suggest that it may regulate the production of proinflammatory cytokines, such as TNF, and serve to direct the clonal expansion of T_H cells.

Possible cytokine regulation by IL-4

Transforming Growth Factor–β

Transforming growth factor (TGF)-β is secreted in active form predominantly by activated T cells and mononuclear phagocytes.[13] It may variably inhibit or promote the growth of a variety of cell types and promote angiogenesis. Transforming growth factor–β inhibits T-cell proliferation to a number of stimuli as well as the maturation of cytotoxic T lymphocytes. Additionally, TGF-β may downregulate the production and activity of the more potent proinflammatory species, thereby serving as a suppressor of immune responses.

Lymphotoxin

Lymphotoxin (LT) is secreted by activated T lymphocytes, often in conjunction with IFN-γ.[14] Interestingly, this cytokine shares a degree of structural homology with TNF (as a result, it is often referred to as TNF-β) and competes with TNF for binding to the same receptors. Although the postreceptor functional responses to LT resemble those of TNF, this cytokine is produced in lesser quantities and probably serves only a local, rather than systemic purpose. In this regard it is an activator of neutrophils and vascular endothelial cells.

MEDIATOR INTERACTIONS FOR MODULATING THE SPECIFIC IMMUNE RESPONSE

Mediators of Specific Immunity

$CD4^+$ T_H1 cells respond to bacteria, protozoa, and viruses

$CD4^+$ T_H2 cells respond to metazoa and allergens

The recognition of different types of pathogens by the specific immune system can result in qualitatively and quantitatively different immune responses. For example, $CD4^+$ T_H1 cells appear to respond primarily to bacteria, protozoa, and viruses whereas $CD4^+$ T_H2 cells respond preferentially to metazoa and allergens.[15] When activated, $CD4^+$ T_H1 cells produce IL-2 and IFN-γ whereas $CD4^+$ T_H2 cells produce IL-4, IL-5, and IL-10.[16,17] Thus, the cytokine profile generated can vary with the type of infecting pathogen.

The mechanism underlying this differential responsiveness of T_H1 and T_H2 cells is not currently known, but implies an additional type of cognition by the immune system. However, it is known that the generation of a T_H1 and T_H2 response is closely controlled by monocyte/macrophage cytokines and cytokines produced by the T_H1 and T_H2 cells themselves. Interleukin-12, TNF, and IL-1 derived from monocytes and macrophages, and IFN-γ derived from NK and T_H1 cells upregulate T_H1 cells and downregulate T_H2 cells. By contrast, monocyte/macrophage IL-10 and IL-6 and T_H2 IL-4, IL-5, and IL-10 upregulate T_H2 cells and downregulate T_H1 cells. Thus, because the cytokines produced by one subset upregulate that subset while downregulating the dichotomous subset, an inertia develops wherein, once the T_H1 or T_H2 response begins to predominate it amplifies itself while inhibiting the opposing response.

Cytokine response to injury

As mentioned previously, empiric data have shown that T_H1 responses predominate in bacterial, viral, and protozoan infections while T_H2 responses do so in metazoan and allergic conditions. As will be discussed in more detail later, the cytokine profile in response to injury suggests that a predisposition for T_H2 responses occurs following injury. Certainly a T_H2 response to injury would appear to be dysfunctional as it would leave the host poorly prepared to deal with subsequent bacterial or viral challenges. One reason the T_H2 responses may be inefficient, particularly against bacterial infections, is that they induce B-lymphocyte class switching such that the immunoglobulin (Ig) G1 (murine) and IgG4 (human) isotypes and IgE predominate.[16] Immunoglobulin G4 and IgE are not able to fix complement, and evidence suggests they also are among the least efficient opsonizing antibodies.[18] Because complement fixation (for subsequent lysis or phagocyte adhesion) and antibody opsonization (for enhanced phagocytosis) are major host defenses against bacteria, a predominant T_H2 response to injury with associated class switching to the IgG4 isotope and IgE would leave the host susceptible to bacterial infections.

T_H2 responses leave host vulnerable to infection

Injury-related decrease in IL-2 and IFN-γ

Injury leads to a deficiency in the production of IL-2 and IFN-γ, a fact established by the direct measurement of these cytokines and documentation of decreased T-cell proliferation in response to mitogens and antigens (which is dependent on IL-2) and a decreased monocyte/macrophage expression of class II MHC molecules (which is dependent, in part, on IFN-γ).[19-21] It is likely that the injury-associated decline in monocyte/macrophage class II MHC molecules also contributes to defective T-cell proliferation. The level of monocyte/macrophage expression of class II MHC molecules is an important factor in the ability of these cells to present antigen in a class II–restricted fashion to $CD4^+$ T cells. Interleukin-2 and IFN-γ are important modulating cytokines for the development of T_H1 and T_H2 responses: they enhance T_H1 responses while inhibiting T_H2 responses. Thus, the resultant decrease in IL-2 and IFN-γ following injury appears to favor development along the T_H2 pathway.

The detection of some proinflammatory cytokines (eg, TNF, IL-1) is not consistently demonstrable following injury alone, in contrast to their detection following infection. It has been proposed that the failure to detect these cytokines systemically does not rule out the possibility of their increased production at the tissue level. Nonetheless, based on current evidence, the production of bioactive forms of these cytokines does not increase consistently following injury. Because increased levels of TNF and IL-1 are associated with T_H1 responses, the failure to consistently detect these cytokines following injury would imply a lack of T_H1 activity. Unlike IL-2 and IFN-γ, TNF and IL-1 do not appear to actively downregulate T_H2 responses, but do directly contribute to the development of T_H1 responses.[9]

Minimal TNF and IL-1 response to injury

Interleukin-4, a major product of the T_H2 cells, plays an important role in the upregulation of T_H2 responses and the downregulation of T_H1 responses. Unfortunately, there are minimal data concerning the effect of injury on this cytokine although it has been shown that inflammation caused by exposure to ultraviolet radiation leads to a T_H2 cytokine profile (increased levels of IL-4 and decreased levels of IL-2 and IFN-γ). However, it also has been shown in vivo and in vitro that gluco-

Glucocorticoids and injury

Glucocorticoids downregulate IL-2 and inhibit IFN-γ, TNF, and IL-1

corticoids (GCs) potently upregulate IL-4 and, as has been demonstrated previously, potently downregulate IL-2.[22,23] Based on this cytokine profile, increased levels of GCs apparently favor T_H2-type responses. Certainly, plasma levels of GCs are elevated following injury. In fact, GC levels may be elevated for weeks following a major injury.[24,25] Additionally, levels of the plasma GC binding proteins, corticosteroid-binding globulin and albumin, are decreased significantly following major injuries, leading to chronic increases in the levels of free, biologically active GCs that may be as many as ten times higher than normal.[26] Under these conditions of GC excess, IL-2 production should be strongly downregulated, as has been demonstrated following injury. Additionally, IL-4 production should be upregulated, although this has yet to be shown definitively. Finally, GCs are known to inhibit the elaboration of IFN-γ, TNF, and IL-1, and this is indeed the profile observed following injury. Thus, chronic elevations of GC levels, as observed in humans who experience a major injury, may be a key regulatory element in directing the specific immune system preferentially to T_H2 rather than T_H1 responsiveness.

IL-10 and IL-12: Key elements in the control of T_H1 and T_H2 responses

Interleukin-12 and IL-10 also are key elements in the control of T_H1 and T_H2 responses. Interleukin-12 appears to be a potent inducer of T_H1 development and an equally potent inhibitor of T_H2 development. By contrast, IL-10 works in an opposite fashion, upregulating T_H2 and downregulating T_H1 responses. Unfortunately, sufficient data are not available concerning the effects of injury on these recently characterized cytokines.

IL-6: A marker for T_H2 cell activation

While IL-6 does not appear to be a major regulatory element in T_H1 vis-à-vis T_H2 responses, it nonetheless is a marker for T_H2 cell activation.[27] Further, IL-6 is one of the few cytokines whose levels have been shown consistently to be elevated systemically following injury and sepsis.[28,29] Levels of IL-6 also have been shown to correlate with the magnitude of underlying injury and physiologic status. Given that IL-6 is a cytokine marker of T_H2 cells, these data provide further evidence for the predominance of the T_H2 pathway following injury.

NATURALLY OCCURRING CYTOKINE ANTAGONISTS

Endogenously derived factors also exert an inhibitory function against many cytokines. These naturally occurring inhibitory proteins have been identified in both the urine and serum of patients with febrile illnesses and malignancies. The recent isolation and cloning of polypeptides directed against the specific activities of TNF and IL-1 defines the existence of additional levels for specific cytokine regulation.[30]

TNF inhibitory proteins

The proteins recently identified as inhibiting TNF activity have been characterized as two distinct species whose molecular weights are approximately 30 and 40 kD. Sequence analysis of these proteins has revealed them to be the extracellular domains of p55 and p75 TNF receptors, respectively. Although the mechanisms for the regulation of these soluble TNF receptor (sTNFr) proteins are still poorly defined, they appear to be shed from the cell surface in response to many of the same inflammatory stimuli that induce TNF production.

The circulating half-life of the sTNFr proteins appears to be short, approximately 20 minutes. The native forms of the proteins, as well as those bound with TNF, are eliminated rapidly through the kidneys. Hence, the appearance of these extracellular TNF binding proteins may be closely linked with conditions in which excessive TNF production occurs or is sustained. Recent data suggest that the presence of such sTNFr proteins may serve to diminish the cytotoxicity of endogenously produced TNF.[31] It is likely that the shedding of cytokine receptors is a common mechanism for the local regulation of specific cytokine activity.

Competitive IL-1α and IL-1β receptor binding protein

In contrast to soluble cytokine receptors and their inhibitory effects, a uniquely different inhibitory protein directed against IL-1 has been identified.[32] The glycosylated form of the inhibitor competes with IL-1α and IL-1β for binding to the cell surface receptor. The recombinant species, an IL-1ra, has been identified widely in a number of inflammatory conditions and has been shown to be effective in the prevention of the cardiovascular collapse attending bacteremia when a 100- to 1,000-time molar excess of IL-1ra over endogenous levels of IL-1 is achieved by exogenous infusion.[33]

CLINICAL STUDIES OF CYTOKINES AND ANTAGONISTS IN SEPSIS AND CRITICAL ILLNESS

Studies in Endotoxemic Humans

Figure 2A

The administration of lipopolysaccharide to otherwise healthy subjects provides an opportunity to elicit cytokine influences under controlled conditions.[34] Numerous investigators have utilized this clinical model of mild inflammation to describe the hemodynamic, immunologic, and metabolic consequences of abbreviated endotoxemia in humans. The results of such studies have corroborated those of animal studies wherein a monophasic appearance of cytokines follows lipopolysaccharide exposure (Fig. 2A). Furthermore, the temporal appearance of cytokines correlates with the acute clinical symptomatology observed in endotoxemic patients. While some early events, such as relative neutropenia, precede the systemic appearance of TNF or other cytokines, other systemic manifestations, such as fever, tachycardia, and increased energy expenditure occur simultaneously with, or subsequent to, detectable cytokinemia.

Catecholamines and cortisol complicating the identification of cytokine-specific stress responses

The counterregulatory stress hormone response to lipopolysaccharide administration complicates the identification of cytokine-specific parameters. For example, catecholamine levels increase within 2 hours of lipopolysaccharide administration, nearly coincident with the appearance of TNF activity. While such a catecholamine response may mimic several hemodynamic and metabolic parameters observed during endotoxemia, this adrenergic discharge dissipates prior to any pyrogenic and energy expenditure manifestations. Hypercortisolemia occurring 2 to 4 hours after lipopolysaccharide administration further complicates the interpretation of cytokine-directed injury responses (Fig. 2A). Although this adrenocortical response exerts little influence upon host hemodynamic processes, this component of the counterregulatory response may direct some aspects of postlipopolysaccharide immune response, such as lymphopenia. The anti-inflammatory nature of the GCs also may serve to dampen or downregulate any tendency toward subsequent cytokine production. This characteristic of the stress cortisol response may serve the teleologically essential function of protecting the host against subsequent cytokine activity should ongoing or repeated endotoxemic challenges occur.

Responses to lipopolysaccharide administration

The responses to lipopolysaccharide administration in normal subjects are remarkably similar to those observed in humans administered recombinant cytokines.[35,36] The host response to TNF or IL-1 administration differs from the lipopolysaccharide challenge primarily in its shorter interval preceding the onset of systemic manifestations. However, the interpretation of cytokine-specific responses is likewise confounded by the attendant stress hormonal milieu arising from the cytokine challenge. Resolution of the specific contributions of cytokines and other hormonal mediators necessitates studies directed toward attenuation of the activities of the individual cytokines.

As noted previously, recent investigations have confirmed that an additional level of cytokine control may be exerted by endogenously derived antagonists. This is particularly true for TNF and IL-1. Recent data have identified the appearance of naturally occurring cytokine antagonists in the forms of soluble receptor

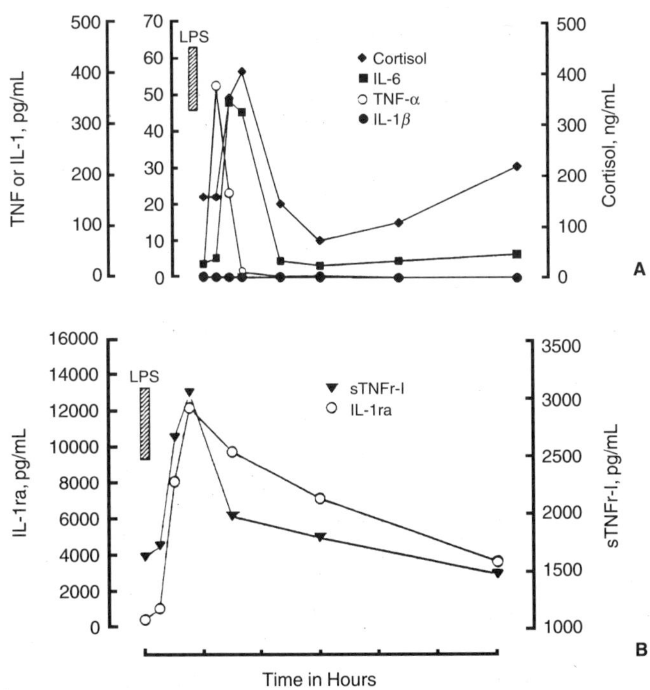

Fig. 2. Levels of **(A)** TNF-α, IL-1β, IL-6, and cortisol and **(B)** sTNFr-I and IL-1ra following the administration of lipopolysaccharide in normal patients. (From Rogy et al.[29] Reprinted with permission.)

Figure 2B

species and receptor antagonists (Fig. 2B) as well as anti-inflammatory cytokines, such as IL-10, during experimental endotoxemia. Our understanding of the balance between proinflammatory mediator activities and those of an anti-inflammatory nature is far too preliminary to yield firm conclusions regarding their absolute activity during the early or later stages of severe infection. However, it appears that a significant proportion of the natural antagonist response is engendered by activities of the proinflammatory cytokines.

Studies in Critically Ill Patients

The clinical spectrum exhibited by infected patients extends from abbreviated episodes of endotoxemia to the more protracted conditions elicited by chronic inflammation or repeated episodes of bacteremia. Although a single episode of septic decompensation may portend a high morbidity, modern principles of clinical management and organ support limit the likelihood of rapid demise. Rather, it is the late sequelae of such events, including the progressive deterioration of organ function, that exacts the highest toll in critical care settings. In many cases the source of the offending organism remains elusive while immunologic and metabolic competence continues to fail. This latter scenario represents a failure of endogenous response mechanisms as well as the available technology to attenuate an infectious insult that, by most quantitative measures, should otherwise be a survivable challenge.

A failure of immunologic and metabolic response mechanisms

As already discussed, cytokine mediators are widely assumed to exert acute pathophysiologic influences in septic and critically ill patients.[31] Among the cytokines exhibiting significant proinflammatory characteristics, TNF and IL-1 appear to be the most promising for promoting the acute septic responses and organ failure sequelae of sepsis. However, several prospective studies that have sought to determine the incidence of TNF and IL-1 detection in critically ill patients have failed to consistently identify these cytokines during clinical conditions consistent with their known biologic functions.

The search for the cytokines of sepsis and multiple organ failure

Although recent studies have suggested that these cytokines may be detectable over prolonged periods in some patients dying

Table 3. Detectable Cytokine Levels* in Patients With Sepsis

	Assay Method	Proportion of Subjects With Detectable Levels		Cytokine Levels	
				Survivors	Nonsurvivors
TNF	Variable	252/514	(49%)	33–840 pg/mL	217–830 pg/mL
IL-1	Variable	70/185	(38%)	153–447 pg/mL	93–1,630 pg/mL
IL-6	7TD1/B.9 hybridoma	113/149	(76%)	25–638 U/mL	270–15,205 U/mL

*Mean or, preferably, median values where available.
(From Lowry et al.[34] Reprinted with permission.)

Table 3

of infection, the general incidence of TNF detection is less than 50% in such patients, and that of IL-1 is even lower (Table 3).[34] Several factors, including a short circulating half-life and episodic production, could account for the low frequency of detection of these proteins. An additional characteristic of these proinflammatory cytokines is their compartmentalized production within tissues. Hence, a significant degree of cytokine activity may exist without the detection of circulating forms. This characteristic is further complicated by a polymorphism that, as documented for TNF and IL-1, provides for biologic activity exerted by cell-associated species.

Little doubt, but little proof, of the role of proinflammatory cytokines in overwhelming bacteremia

Currently there is little doubt regarding the participation of one or more proinflammatory cytokines in the acute hemodynamic collapse attending many cases of severe endotoxemia or bacteremia. However, there is no evidence of the participation of these cytokines beyond the earliest phases of the sepsis syndrome. The levels of cytokinemia observed following the onset of sepsis are seldom significantly different from those achieved in response to an abbreviated lipopolysaccharide challenge, suggesting that the level of initial activation is not sufficient to sustain the full spectrum of observed endotoxemic or bacteremic clinical responses. To some extent the mechanistic dilemma presented by this failure to frequently detect free cytokine levels during sepsis is resolved by evidence that much of the activity of these cytokines occurs at the tissue level. In addition, there are data to suggest their presence in association with binding proteins. Nevertheless, a paucity of data exists to support the concept of a prolonged and/or excessive bioactivity of these cytokines within tissues. This, coupled with the potential for attenuation of the cytokines' activity through endogenous components of the stress hormone response, suggests that their activity may be episodic. There can be little doubt regarding the participation of the proinflammatory cytokines in the acute hemodynamic collapse attending many cases of overwhelming bacteremia.

An unclear relationship between cytokines and multiple organ failure

It is within the more protracted clinical sequelae of infection and injury that cytokine-induced pathology is most conceptually alluring, and yet difficult to document. While a tendency toward an increased incidence of cytokinemia in the presence of organ failure has been noted, the causal relationship of such findings to the progression of multiple organ failure remains unclear.[37] Here, too, the level of cytokinemia frequently observed in patients with multiple-system organ failure is seldom greater than that noted in patients following a survivable lipopolysaccharide or bacterial challenge. Additionally, the impact of chronic cytokinemia upon the normal capacity for receptor-ligand binding and signal transduction remains undefined.

Endogenous antagonist production and activity further complicates the assignment of cytokine-specific activity during the more chronic phases of infection. While sTNFrs and IL-1ra are inducible by endotoxin administration, a generally similar level of sTNFr and IL-1ra species can be identified in patients with severe bacterial infection. Recently we have sought to determine the relationship between critical illness and the presence of the proinflammatory cytokines TNF and IL-1 and their natural antagonists.[29] We studied a consecutive series of patients who were admitted to a critical care unit because of major injury or infection. At the time of admission the incidence of TNF and IL-1 detection was exceedingly low (Fig. 3). Despite these findings, there was a much higher incidence of IL-6, sTNFr, and IL-1ra detection. Whereas the levels of some cytokines (eg, IL-6) correlated roughly with the magnitude of underlying injury and physiologic status, no clear relationship existed for the presence of circulating TNF or IL-1 nor for their respective antagonists. It is of interest that the levels of such natural cytokine antagonists do not reflect the severity of the inciting challenge nor initial clinical presentation. Hence, circulating levels of natural cytokine antagonists appear less responsive to the magnitude of the insult than do other components of the stress hormone response.

Figure 3

PRELIMINARY RESULTS FROM CLINICAL TRIALS OF ANTICYTOKINE THERAPIES

Clinical studies utilizing a variety of anticytokine therapies have been initiated during the past several years.[38] Currently several prospective trials are evaluating the response to TNF blockade utilizing various antibody constructs directed against this cytokine (Table 4), including a recently reported phase II trial of a murine IgG.[39] The preliminary results of a recent phase III trial have been presented in abbreviated format,[40] but it appears that such agents have relatively little impact on long-term survival except in patients who are in septic shock at the time they seek medical help. As might be anticipated, a recent report of one such anti-TNF agent suggests that improved biologic responses are

Table 4

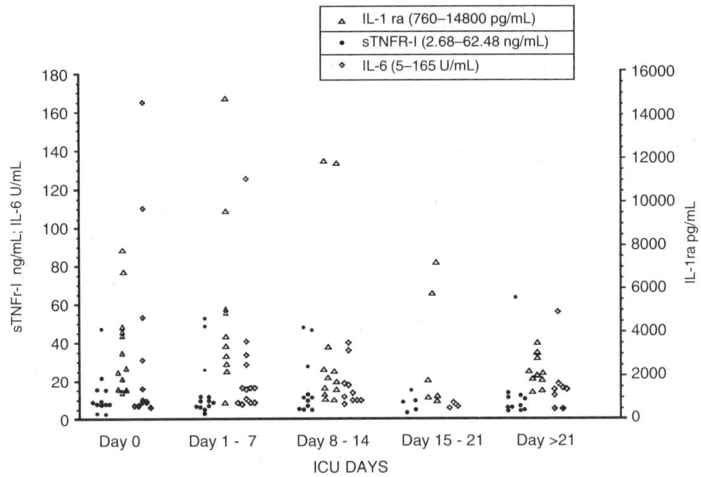

Fig. 3. Levels of sTNFr-I, IL-1ra, and IL-6 in critically ill patients with sepsis syndrome. (From Rogy et al.[29] Reprinted with permission.)

more readily observed when circulating TNF is detectable at the outset of therapy.[39]

Investigating competitive TNF-receptor binding proteins

An additional strategy currently under investigation to reduce TNF activity involves the use of soluble TNF receptor constructs (immunoadhesions) of the p55 and p75 receptors. These are unique molecules that combine two extracellular receptor components in fusion with the Fc portion of IgG. In theory, such constructs enhance ligand binding and increase the biologic half-lives of the antagonists. At the time of this writing a phase II (p55) trial is currently under way and a phase II (p75) trial has recently been completed.

Trials of IL-1 receptor antagonist in septic patients

Also recently completed was a phase III trial of IL-1ra intervention in septic patients.[41] The authors did not observe a statistically significant correlation with prospective 28-day all-cause mortality, nor did they note a statistical improvement in survival based upon prospectively defined criteria for shock at study entry. However, a retrospective analysis of the data based upon a risk-prediction model was proposed to demonstrate a benefit of the antagonist in patients at increased risk for in-hospital mortality. In this analysis, IL-1ra therapy also appeared to improve 28-day mortality in patients presenting with sepsis-associated organ dysfunction or shock. However, a recent phase III trial of IL-1ra using shock and/or organ dysfunction as end points was discontinued after interim analysis failed to reproduce this apparent benefit.

IMPLICATIONS FOR CYTOKINE ANTAGONIST THERAPY

A wealth of preclinical data suggests that the acute attenuation of TNF and IL-1 activities represents a desirable therapeutic objective in some critically ill patients. Nevertheless, there is also evidence to suggest that a lack of such cytokine activity may portend poorly in some stressed patients. The clinical observations in support of this theory frequently have been made in

Table 4. Tumor Necrosis Factor–α Antagonists Currently Under Clinical Development

Sponsor	TNF-α Antagonist	Study Phase
Celltech		
CB0006	Murine IgG	II
CDP571	Humanized mouse IgG	III
Bayer-Miles	Murine IgG	III
Centocor	Mouse chimeric IgG	II
Immunex	Human dimeric sTNFr	II
Hoffmann-LaRoche	Human dimeric sTNFr	II

(From Suffredini.[38] Reprinted with permission.)

patients who remain critically ill for extended periods and experience an attendant deterioration of nutritional status and organ system function. This is in contrast to what is seen in patients during the first hours or days following acute injury or invasive infection. Hence, it is likely that the earlier events are more susceptible to a brief period of cytokine antagonist therapy. It has been hypothesized that this acute anticytokine therapy serves to dampen the subsequent inflammatory response.

Most effective time for cytokine antagonist therapy

The more prolonged recovery and tissue repair phases may require some cytokine activity to proceed in a normal fashion. The abbreviated nature of the counterregulatory stress hormone response as well as the short biologic half-lives of the naturally occurring cytokine antagonists may indirectly testify to such a necessity. Hence, any tendency to extend anticytokine therapies beyond the early flow phase of injury must be addressed experimentally before such therapies can be implemented clinically. Although current clinical investigation is directed toward the acute attenuation of cytokine activity, such therapeutic strategies might, if improperly timed or excessive, serve to alter a teleologically delicate balance between the beneficial influence of modest cytokine activity and the acutely adverse consequences of excessive cytokine influences.

Balancing beneficial and adverse cytokine influences

References

1. Vassalli P, in Paul WE, et al (eds). *Annual Review of Immunology*, vol 10. Palo Alto, Calif, Annual Reviews Inc, 1992, pp 411-452.
2. Tracey KJ, et al. *Science* 1986;234:470-474.
3. Dinarello CA. *Immunol Rev* 1992;127:119-146.
4. Eisenberg SP, et al. *Nature* 1990;343:341-346.
5. Gauldio J, et al. *Res Immunol* 1992;143:755-759.
6. Yoshimura T, et al. *Proc Natl Acad Sci USA* 1987;84:9233-9237.
7. Howard M, O'Garra A. *Immunol Today* 1992;13:198-200.
8. Moore KW, et al, in Paul WE, et al (eds). *Annual Review of Immunology*, vol 11. Palo Alto, Calif, Annual Review Inc, 1993, pp 165-190.
9. Trinchieri G. *Immunol Today* 1993;14:335-337.
10. Scott P. *Science* 1993;206:496-497.
11. Kirchner H, Marcucci F, in Vilcek J, DeMaeyer E (eds). *Interferon 2: Interferons and the Immune System*. Amsterdam, Elsevier, 1984, pp 7-34.
12. Robb RJ. *Immunol Today* 1984;5:203-209.
13. Wahl SM, et al. *Immunol Today* 1989;10:258-261.
14. Pennica D, et al. *Nature* 1984;312:724-729.
15. Scott P, Kaufmann SHE. *Immunol Today* 1991;12:346-348.
16. Möller G (ed). *Immunological Reviews*, vol 123. Copenhagen, Munksgaard, 1991, pp 5-229.
17. Romagnami S. *Immunol Today* 1991;12:256-257.
18. Morrison SL, in Paul WE, et al (eds). *Annual Review of Immunology*, vol 10. Palo Alto, Calif, Annual Reviews Inc, 1992, pp 248-249.
19. Wood JJ, et al. *Ann Surg* 1984;200:311-320.
20. Hershman MJ, et al. *Clin Exp Immunol* 1989;77:67-70.
21. Hershman MJ, et al. *Br J Surg* 1990;77:204-207.
22. Daynes RA, Araneo BA. *Eur J Immunol* 1989;19:2319-2325.
23. Daynes RA, et al. *J Exp Med* 1990;171:979-996.
24. Vaughn GM, et al. *J Trauma* 1982;22:263-273.
25. Calvano SE, et al. *J Burn Care Rehab* 1984;5:143-151.
26. Murray D. *J Endocrinol* 1967;39:571-591.
27. Mosmann TR, et al. *J Immunol* 1986;136:2348-2357.
28. Fong Y, et al. *Surg Gynecol Obstet* 1990;170:363-378.

29. Rogy MA, et al. *J Am Coll Surg* 1994;178:132-138.
30. Fong Y, Lowry SF, in Wilmore DW, et al (eds). *Care of the Surgical Patient*, vol 1. New York, NY, Scientific American, sect 4, chap 7, 1990, pp 1-17.
31. Lowry SF, Moldawer LL, in Vincent J-L (ed). *Yearbook of Intensive Care and Emergency Medicine, Update 1992*. Berlin, Springer-Verlag, 1992, pp 36-43.
32. Dinarello CA. *J Infect Dis* 1991;163:1177-1184.
33. Fischer E, et al. *J Clin Invest* 1992;89:1551-1557.
34. Lowry SF, et al, in Vincent JL (ed). *Yearbook of Intensive Care and Emergency Medicine 1994*. Berlin, Springer-Verlag, 1994, pp 14-23.
35. van der Poll T, Lowry SF, in Tellado JM (ed). *Modulation of the Inflammatory Response in Severe Sepsis*. Basel, Karger Editorial, in press.
36. van der Poll T, et al. *N Engl J Med* 1990;322:1622-1627.
37. Lowry SF. *Soc Crit Care Med* 1993;1:120-126.
38. Suffredini AF. *Crit Care Med*, in press.
39. Fisher CJ, et al. *Crit Care Med* 1993;21:318-327.
40. Wherry J, et al. *Chest* 1993;104:3S.
41. Fisher CJ, et al. *JAMA* 1994;271:1836-1843.

Index

Page numbers in **boldface** type refer to pages on which tables or figures appear; an *italic t* or *f* denotes tables or figures, respectively.

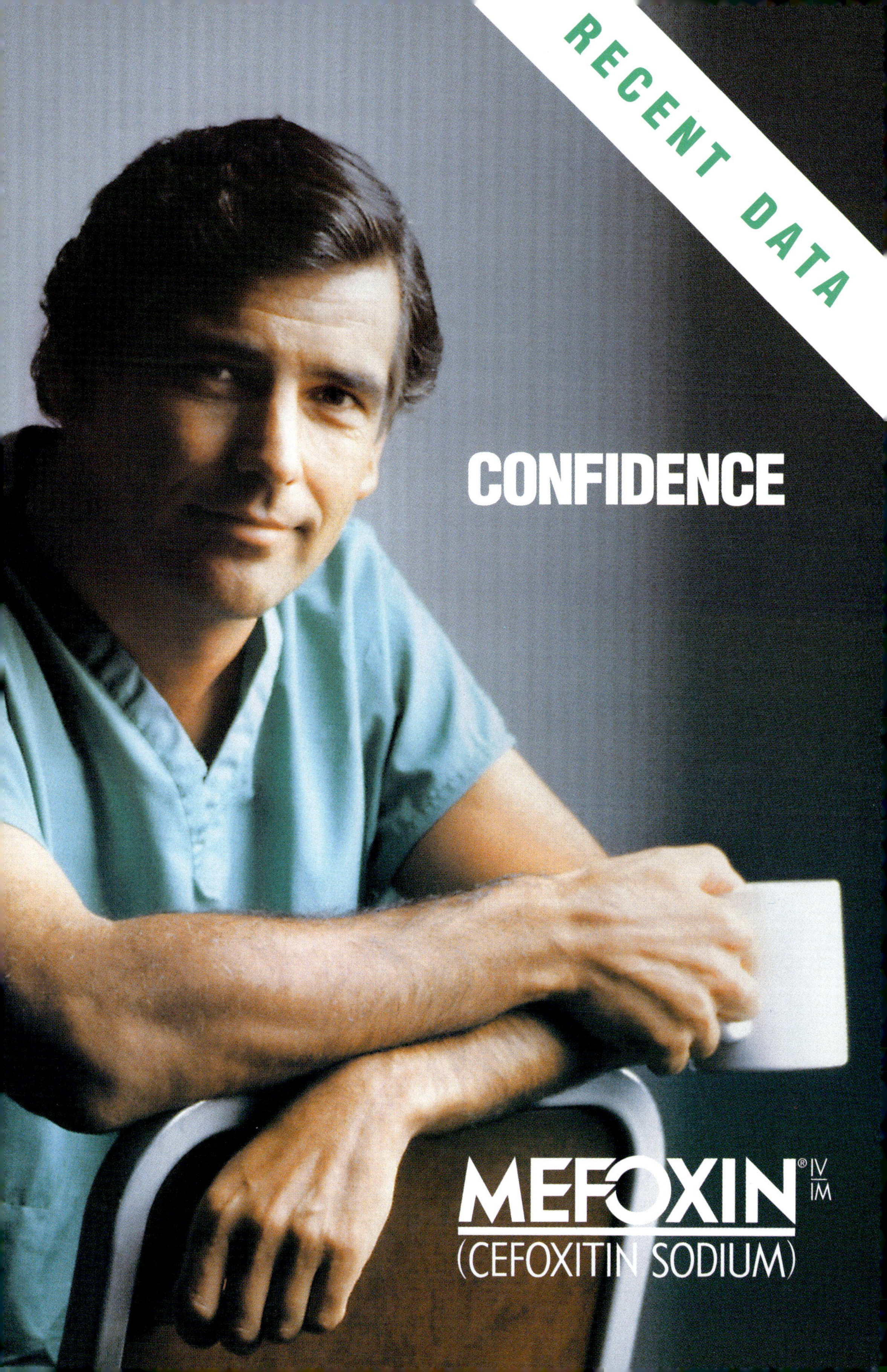
RECENT DATA
CONFIDENCE
MEFOXIN® IV/IM
(CEFOXITIN SODIUM)

In a recent study of penetrating abdominal trauma, 144 patients (85% of total) were categorized in group 1 (low risk) and had 2 days of antibiotic therapy; 26 patients (15% of total) were categorized as group 2 or group 3 (mid or high risk) and received 5 days of antibiotic therapy.[1]

MORE EFFECTIVE THAN CEFOTAN* IN LOW-RISK PATIENTS**

...in preventing infection in 2-day therapy group

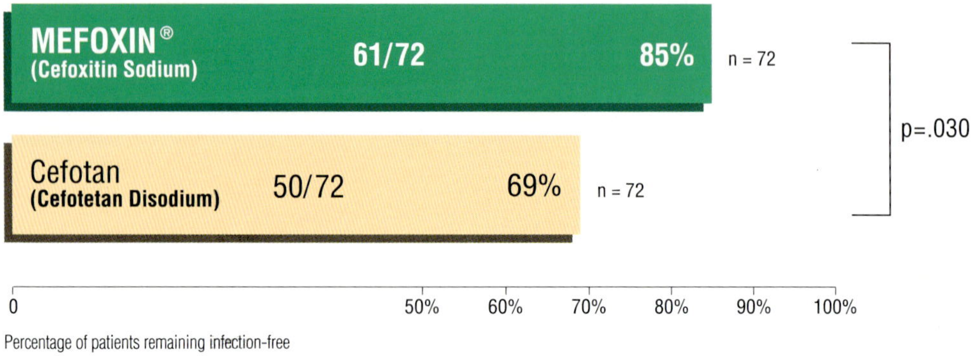

...in significantly reducing length of hospital stay in 2-day, low-risk therapy group

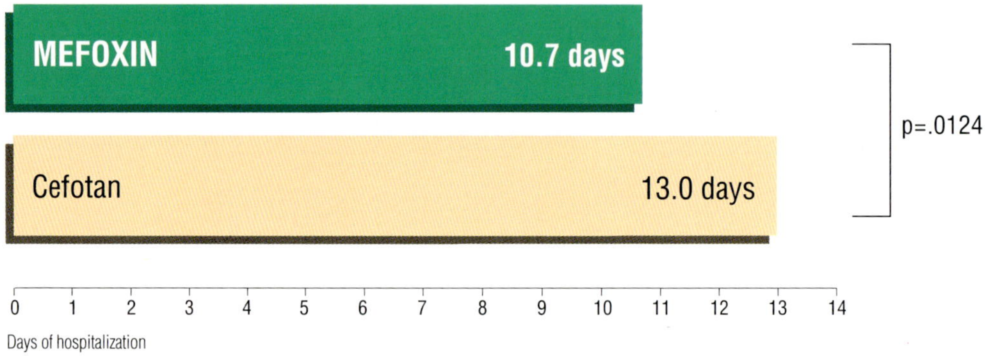

* registered trademark of Imperial Chemical Industries PLC for cefotetan disodium

** In mid- to high-risk patients treated for 5 days, length of hospitalization was almost twice as long for cefoxitin-treated patients than for those treated with cefotetan (p=.037), while infections prevented were 47% and 36% for cefoxitin and cefotetan, respectively.

The prophylactic administration of MEFOXIN may reduce the incidence of certain postoperative infections in patients undergoing surgical procedures (e.g., hysterectomy, gastrointestinal surgery, and transurethral prostatectomy) that are classified as contaminated or potentially contaminated.

Pseudomembranous colitis, from mild to life-threatening in severity, has been reported with virtually all antibiotics (including cephalosporins); therefore, it is important to consider its diagnosis when diarrhea develops in association with antibiotic use.

1. Adapted from *Arch. Surg.*, 1993; 128:55-64

In an *in vitro** study by Goldstein and Citron[2]

A comparison of anaerobic coverage vs. Cefotan

***In vitro* susceptibilities of isolates from two community hospitals at a 32-mcg/mL breakpoint (n=215)[2]**

	*B. fragilis***	*B. thetaiota-omicron*	*B. distasonis*	*B. vulgatus*	*B. ovatus*
MEFOXIN	**97%**	**92%**	**69%**	**93%**	**82%**
Cefotan	93%	24%	16%	93%	12%

** NOTE: Based on the 1994 *Physicians' Desk Reference®*, Cefotan is usually active *in vitro* and in clinical infections against a number of organisms, including *Bacteroides* species (excluding *B. distasonis*, *B. ovatus*, and *B. thetaiotaomicron*).

MEFOXIN is contraindicated in patients who have shown hypersensitivity to cefoxitin and the cephalosporin group of antibiotics.

Before therapy with MEFOXIN is instituted, careful inquiry should be made to determine whether the patient has had previous hypersensitivity reactions to cefoxitin, cephalosporins, penicillins, or other drugs. This product should be given with caution to penicillin-sensitive patients. Antibiotics should be administered with caution to any patient who has demonstrated some form of allergy, particularly to drugs. If an allergic reaction to MEFOXIN occurs, discontinue the drug. Serious hypersensitivity reactions may require epinephrine and other emergency measures.

* The clinical significance of these *in vitro* data has not been established.

2. Goldstein, E.J.C. and Citron, D.M., *J. Clin. Microbiol.*, 1988

BALANCED COVERAGE† WITH

MEFOXIN® IV/IM

(CEFOXITIN SODIUM)

† Denotes *in vitro* activity against indicated aerobes and anaerobes. This does not necessarily imply clinical efficacy.

An Antibiotic of Choice*...

FOR SIGNIFICANT MEDICAL REASONS

- Clinical experience in over 19 million patients**
- Balanced *in vitro* coverage of many important aerobes and anaerobes
- Specific pediatric dosage guidelines***

FOR SIGNIFICANT ECONOMIC REASONS

- Competitively priced

See your Merck Representative for a discussion of the potential value of MEFOXIN to your patients and to your hospital.

* For the treatment of indicated bacterial infections at indicated sites.

** Estimate based on total usage in the United States.

*** Safety and efficacy in infants from birth to 3 months of age have not yet been established.

Please read the accompanying full Prescribing Information before prescribing.

BALANCED COVERAGE† WITH

MEFOXIN® IV/IM
(CEFOXITIN SODIUM)

† Denotes *in vitro* activity against indicated aerobes and anaerobes. This does not necessarily imply clinical efficacy.

The most common adverse reactions have been local reactions following intravenous injection.

1. Nichols, R. L. et al.: Prospective alterations in therapy for penetrating abdominal trauma, Arch. Surg. *128*:55-64, January 1993.
2. Goldstein, E.J.C. and Citron, D.M.: Annual incidence, epidemiology, and comparative in vitro susceptibilities to cefoxitin, cefotetan, cefmetazole, and ceftizoxime of recent community-acquired isolates of the *Bacteroides fragilis* group, J. Clin. Microbiol. *26(11)*:2361-2366, November 1988.

MERCK

MEFOXIN®

(STERILE CEFOXITIN SODIUM)

DESCRIPTION

MEFOXIN† (Sterile Cefoxitin Sodium) is a semi-synthetic, broad-spectrum cepha antibiotic sealed under nitrogen for parenteral administration. It is derived from cephamycin C, which is produced by *Streptomyces lactamdurans*. It is the sodium salt of 3-(hydroxymethyl)-7α-methoxy-8-oxo-7-[2-(2-thienyl)acetamido]-5-thia-1-azabicyclo [4.2.0] oct-2-ene-2-carboxylate carbamate (ester). The empirical formula is $C_{16}H_{16}N_3NaO_7S_2$, and the structural formula is:

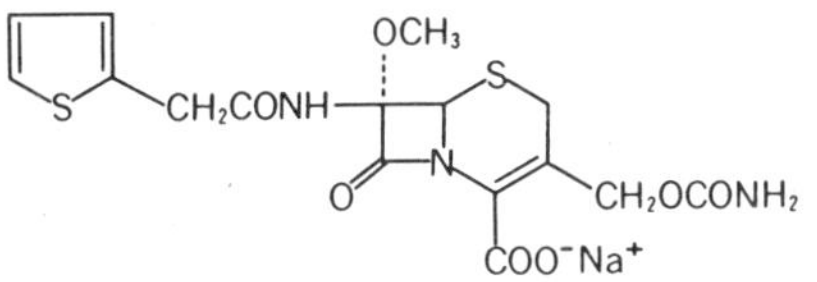

MEFOXIN contains approximately 53.8 mg (2.3 milliequivalents) of sodium per gram of cefoxitin activity. Solutions of MEFOXIN range from colorless to light amber in color. The pH of freshly constituted solutions usually ranges from 4.2 to 7.0.

CLINICAL PHARMACOLOGY

Clinical Pharmacology

After intramuscular administration of a 1 gram dose of MEFOXIN to normal volunteers, the mean peak serum concentration was 24 mcg/mL. The peak occurred at 20 to 30 minutes. Following an intravenous dose of 1 gram, serum concentrations were 110 mcg/mL at 5 minutes, declining to less than 1 mcg/mL at 4 hours. The half-life after an intravenous dose is 41 to 59 minutes; after intramuscular administration, the half-life is 64.8 minutes. Approximately 85 percent of cefoxitin is excreted unchanged by the kidneys over a 6-hour period, resulting in high urinary concentrations. Following an intramuscular dose of 1 gram, urinary concentrations greater than 3000 mcg/mL were observed. Probenecid slows tubular excretion and produces higher serum levels and increases the duration of measurable serum concentrations.

Cefoxitin passes into pleural and joint fluids and is detectable in antibacterial concentrations in bile.

Clinical experience has demonstrated that MEFOXIN can be administered to patients who are also receiving carbenicillin, kanamycin, gentamicin, tobramycin, or amikacin (see PRECAUTIONS and ADMINISTRATION).

Microbiology

The bactericidal action of cefoxitin results from inhibition of cell wall synthesis. Cefoxitin has *in vitro* activity against a wide range of gram-positive and gram-negative organisms. The methoxy group in the 7α position provides MEFOXIN with a high degree of stability in the presence of beta-lactamases, both penicillinases and cephalosporinases, of gram-negative bacteria. Cefoxitin is usually active against the following organisms *in vitro* and in clinical infections:

Gram-positive

Staphylococcus aureus, including penicillinase and non-penicillinase producing strains
Staphylococcus epidermidis
Beta-hemolytic and other streptococci (most strains of enterococci, e.g., *Streptococcus faecalis*, are resistant)
Streptococcus pneumoniae

Gram-negative

Escherichia coli
Klebsiella species (including *K. pneumoniae*)
Hemophilus influenzae
Neisseria gonorrhoeae, including penicillinase and non-penicillinase producing strains
Proteus mirabilis
Morganella morganii
Proteus vulgaris
Providencia species, including *Providencia rettgeri*

Anaerobic organisms

Peptococcus species
Peptostreptococcus species
Clostridium species
Bacteroides species, including the *B. fragilis* group (includes *B. fragilis, B. distasonis, B. ovatus, B. thetaiotaomicron, B. vulgatus*)

MEFOXIN is inactive *in vitro* against most strains of *Pseudomonas aeruginosa* and enterococci and many strains of *Enterobacter cloacae*.

Methicillin-resistant staphylococci are almost uniformly resistant to MEFOXIN.

Susceptibility Tests

For fast-growing aerobic organisms, quantitative methods that require measurements of zone diameters give the most precise estimates of antibiotic susceptibility. One such procedure* has been recommended for use with discs to test susceptibility to cefoxitin. Interpretation involves correlation of the diameters obtained in the disc test with minimal inhibitory concentration (MIC) values for cefoxitin.

Reports from the laboratory giving results of the standardized single disc susceptibility test* using a 30 mcg cefoxitin disc should be interpreted according to the following criteria:

Organisms producing zones of 18 mm or greater are considered susceptible, indicating that the tested organism is likely to respond to therapy.

Organisms of intermediate susceptibility produce zones of 15 to 17 mm, indicating that the tested organism would be susceptible if high dosage is used or if the infection is confined to tissues and fluids (e.g., urine) in which high antibiotic levels are attained.

Resistant organisms produce zones of 14 mm or less, indicating that other therapy should be selected.

The cefoxitin disc should be used for testing cefoxitin susceptibility.

Cefoxitin has been shown by *in vitro* tests to have activity against certain strains of *Enterobacteriaceae* found resistant when tested with the cephalosporin class disc. For this reason, the cefoxitin disc should not be used for testing susceptibility to cephalosporins, and cephalosporin discs should not be used for testing susceptibility to cefoxitin.

Dilution methods, preferably the agar plate dilution procedure, are most accurate for susceptibility testing of obligate anaerobes.

A bacterial isolate may be considered susceptible if the MIC value for cefoxitin** is not more than 16 mcg/mL. Organisms are considered resistant if the MIC is greater than 32 mcg/mL.

INDICATIONS AND USAGE

Treatment

MEFOXIN is indicated for the treatment of serious infections caused by susceptible strains of the designated microorganisms in the diseases listed below.

(1) **Lower respiratory tract infections,** including pneumonia and lung abscess, caused by *Streptococcus pneumoniae*, other streptococci (excluding enterococci, e.g., *Streptococcus faecalis*), *Staphylococcus aureus* (penicillinase and non-penicillinase producing), *Escherichia coli, Klebsiella* species, *Hemophilus influenzae*, and *Bacteroides* species.

(2) **Genitourinary infections.** Urinary tract infections caused by *Escherichia coli, Klebsiella* species, *Proteus mirabilis*, indole-positive Proteus (which include the organisms now called *Morganella morganii* and *Proteus vulgaris*), and *Providencia* species (including *Providencia rettgeri*). Uncomplicated gonorrhea due to *Neisseria gonorrhoeae* (penicillinase and non-penicillinase producing).

(3) **Intra-abdominal infections,** including peritonitis and intra-abdominal abscess, caused by *Escherichia coli, Klebsiella* species, *Bacteroides* species including the *Bacteroides fragilis* group***, and *Clostridium* species.

(4) **Gynecological infections,** including endometritis, pelvic cellulitis, and pelvic inflammatory disease caused by *Escherichia coli, Neisseria gonorrhoeae* (penicillinase and non-penicillinase producing), *Bacteroides* species including the *Bacteroides fragilis* group***, *Clostridium* species, *Peptococcus* species, *Peptostreptococcus* species, and Group B streptococci.

(5) **Septicemia** caused by *Streptococcus pneumoniae, Staphylococcus aureus* (penicillinase and non-penicillinase producing), *Escherichia coli, Klebsiella* species, and *Bacteroides* species including the *Bacteroides fragilis* group.***

(6) **Bone and joint infections** caused by *Staphylococcus aureus* (penicillinase and non-penicillinase producing).

(7) **Skin and skin structure infections** caused by *Staphylococcus aureus* (penicillinase and non-penicillinase producing), *Staphylococcus epidermidis*, streptococci (excluding enterococci e.g., *Streptococcus faecalis*), *Escherichia coli, Proteus mirabilis, Klebsiella* species, *Bacteroides* species including the *Bacteroides fragilis* group***, *Clostridium* species, *Peptococcus* species, and *Peptostreptococcus* species.

Appropriate culture and susceptibility studies should be performed to determine the susceptibility of the causative organisms to MEFOXIN. Therapy may be started while awaiting the results of these studies.

In randomized comparative studies, MEFOXIN and cephalothin were comparably safe and effective in the management of infections caused by gram-positive cocci and gram-negative rods susceptible to the cephalosporins. MEFOXIN has a high degree of stability in the presence of bacterial beta-lactamases, both penicillinases and cephalosporinases.

Many infections caused by aerobic and anaerobic gram-negative bacteria resistant to some cephalosporins respond to MEFOXIN. Similarly, many infections caused by aerobic and anaerobic bacteria resistant to some penicillin antibiotics (ampicillin, carbenicillin, penicillin G) respond to treatment with MEFOXIN. Many infections caused by mixtures of susceptible aerobic and anaerobic bacteria respond to treatment with MEFOXIN.

*Bauer, A. W.; Kirby, W. M. M.; Sherris, J. C.; Turck, M.: Antibiotic susceptibility testing by a standardized single disc method, Amer. J. Clin. Path. *45:* 493-496, Apr. 1966. Standardized disc susceptibility test, Federal Register *37:* 20527-20529, 1972. National Committee for Clinical Laboratory Standards: Approved Standard: ASM-2, Performance Standards for Antimicrobial Disc Susceptibility Tests, July 1975.

**Determined by the ICS agar dilution method (Ericsson and Sherris, Acta Path. Microbiol. Scand. [B] Suppl. No. 217, 1971) or any other method that has been shown to give equivalent results.

****B. fragilis, B. distasonis, B. ovatus, B. thetaiotaomicron, B. vulgatus.*

Prevention

When compared to placebo in randomized controlled studies in patients undergoing gastrointestinal surgery, vaginal hysterectomy, abdominal hysterectomy and cesarean section, the prophylactic use of MEFOXIN resulted in a significant reduction in the number of postoperative infections.

The prophylactic administration of MEFOXIN may reduce the incidence of certain postoperative infections in patients undergoing surgical procedures (e.g., hysterectomy, gastrointestinal surgery and transurethral prostatectomy) that are classified as contaminated or potentially contaminated.

The perioperative use of MEFOXIN may be effective in surgical patients in whom subsequent infection at the operative site would present a serious risk, e.g., prosthetic arthroplasty.

Effective prophylactic use depends on the time of administration. MEFOXIN usually should be given one-half to one hour before the operation, which is sufficient time to achieve effective levels in the wound during the procedure. Prophylactic administration should usually be stopped within 24 hours since continuing administration of any antibiotic increases the possibility of adverse reactions but, in the majority of surgical procedures, does not reduce the incidence of subsequent infection. However, in patients undergoing prosthetic arthroplasty, it is recommended that MEFOXIN be continued for 72 hours after the surgical procedure.

If there are signs of infection, specimens for culture should be obtained for identification of the causative organism so that appropriate treatment may be instituted.

CONTRAINDICATIONS

MEFOXIN is contraindicated in patients who have shown hypersensitivity to cefoxitin and the cephalosporin group of antibiotics.

WARNINGS

BEFORE THERAPY WITH 'MEFOXIN' IS INSTITUTED, CAREFUL INQUIRY SHOULD BE MADE TO DETERMINE WHETHER THE PATIENT HAS HAD PREVIOUS HYPERSENSITIVITY REACTIONS TO CEFOXITIN, CEPHALOSPORINS, PENICILLINS, OR OTHER DRUGS. THIS PRODUCT SHOULD BE GIVEN WITH CAUTION TO PENICILLIN-SENSITIVE PATIENTS. ANTIBIOTICS SHOULD BE ADMINISTERED WITH CAUTION TO ANY PATIENT WHO HAS DEMONSTRATED SOME FORM OF ALLERGY, PARTICULARLY TO DRUGS. IF AN ALLERGIC REACTION TO 'MEFOXIN' OCCURS, DISCONTINUE THE DRUG. SERIOUS HYPERSENSITIVITY REACTIONS MAY REQUIRE EPINEPHRINE AND OTHER EMERGENCY MEASURES.

Pseudomembranous colitis has been reported with virtually all antibiotics (including cephalosporins); therefore, it is important to consider its diagnosis in patients who develop diarrhea in association with antibiotic use. This colitis may range from mild to life threatening in severity.

Treatment with broad-spectrum antibiotics alters normal flora of the colon and may permit overgrowth of clostridia. Studies indicate a toxin produced by *clostridium difficile* is one primary cause of antibiotic-associated colitis.

Mild cases of pseudomembranous colitis may respond to drug discontinuance alone. In more severe cases, management may include sigmoidoscopy, appropriate bacteriological studies, fluid, electrolyte and protein supplementation, and the use of a drug such as oral vancomycin as indicated. Isolation of the patient may be advisable. Other causes of colitis should also be considered.

PRECAUTIONS

General

The total daily dose should be reduced when MEFOXIN is administered to patients with transient or persistent reduction of urinary output due to renal insufficiency (see DOSAGE), because high and prolonged serum antibiotic concentrations can occur in such individuals from usual doses.

Antibiotics (including cephalosporins) should be prescribed with caution in individuals with a history of gastrointestinal disease, particularly colitis.

As with other antibiotics, prolonged use of MEFOXIN may result in overgrowth of nonsusceptible organisms. Repeated evaluation of the patient's condition is essential. If superinfection occurs during therapy, appropriate measures should be taken.

Drug Interactions

Increased nephrotoxicity has been reported following concomitant administration of cephalosporins and aminoglycoside antibiotics.

Drug/Laboratory Test Interactions

As with cephalothin, high concentrations of cefoxitin (>100 micrograms/mL) may interfere with measurement of serum and urine creatinine levels by the Jaffé reaction, and produce false increases of modest degree in the levels of creatinine reported. Serum samples from patients treated with cefoxitin should not be analyzed for creatinine if withdrawn within 2 hours of drug administration.

High concentrations of cefoxitin in the urine may interfere with measurement of urinary 17-hydroxy-corticosteroids by the Porter-Silber reaction, and produce false increases of modest degree in the levels reported.

A false-positive reaction for glucose in the urine may occur. This has been observed with CLINITEST†† reagent tablets.

††Registered trademark of Ames Company, Division of Miles Laboratories, Inc.

MEFOXIN® (Sterile Cefoxitin Sodium)

Carcinogenesis, Mutagenesis, Impairment of Fertility

Long-term studies in animals have not been performed with cefoxitin to evaluate carcinogenic or mutagenic potential. Studies in rats treated intravenously with 400 mg/kg of cefoxitin (approximately three times the maximum recommended human dose) revealed no effects on fertility or mating ability.

Pregnancy

Pregnancy Category B. Reproduction studies performed in rats and mice at parenteral doses of approximately one to seven and one-half times the maximum recommended human dose did not reveal teratogenic or fetal toxic effects, although a slight decrease in fetal weight was observed.

There are, however, no adequate and well-controlled studies in pregnant women. Because animal reproduction studies are not always predictive of human response, this drug should be used during pregnancy only if clearly needed.

In the rabbit, cefoxitin was associated with a high incidence of abortion and maternal death. This was not considered to be a teratogenic effect but an expected consequence of the rabbit's unusual sensitivity to antibiotic-induced changes in the population of the microflora of the intestine.

Nursing Mothers

MEFOXIN is excreted in human milk in low concentrations. Caution should be exercised when MEFOXIN is administered to a nursing woman.

Pediatric Use

Safety and efficacy in infants from birth to three months of age have not yet been established. In children three months of age and older, higher doses of MEFOXIN have been associated with an increased incidence of eosinophilia and elevated SGOT.

ADVERSE REACTIONS

MEFOXIN is generally well tolerated. The most common adverse reactions have been local reactions following intravenous or intramuscular injection. Other adverse reactions have been encountered infrequently.

Local Reactions

Thrombophlebitis has occurred with intravenous administration. Pain, induration, and tenderness after intramuscular injections have been reported.

Allergic Reactions

Rash (including exfoliative dermatitis and toxic epidermal necrolysis), pruritus, eosinophilia, fever, dyspnea, and other allergic reactions including anaphylaxis, interstitial nephritis and angioedema have been noted.

Cardiovascular

Hypotension

Gastrointestinal

Diarrhea, including documented pseudomembranous colitis which can appear during or after antibiotic treatment. Nausea and vomiting have been reported rarely.

Neuromuscular

Possible exacerbation of myasthenia gravis

Blood

Eosinophilia, leukopenia including granulocytopenia, neutropenia, anemia, including hemolytic anemia, thrombocytopenia, and bone marrow depression. A positive direct Coombs test may develop in some individuals, especially those with azotemia.

Liver Function

Transient elevations in SGOT, SGPT, serum LDH, and serum alkaline phosphatase; and jaundice have been reported.

Renal Function

Elevations in serum creatinine and/or blood urea nitrogen levels have been observed. As with the cephalosporins, acute renal failure has been reported rarely. The role of MEFOXIN in changes in renal function tests is difficult to assess, since factors predisposing to prerenal azotemia or to impaired renal function usually have been present.

OVERDOSAGE

The acute intravenous LD_{50} in the adult female mouse and rabbit was about 8.0 g/kg and greater than 1.0 g/kg respectively. The acute intraperitoneal LD_{50} in the adult rat was greater than 10.0 g/kg.

DOSAGE

TREATMENT

Adults

The usual adult dosage range is 1 gram to 2 grams every six to eight hours. Dosage and route of administration should be determined by susceptibility of the causative organisms, severity of infection, and the condition of the patient (see Table 1 for dosage guidelines).

MEFOXIN may be used in patients with reduced renal function with the following dosage adjustments:

In adults with renal insufficiency, an initial loading dose of 1 gram to 2 grams may be given. After a loading dose, the recommendations for *maintenance dosage* (Table 2) may be used as a guide.

When only the serum creatinine level is available, the following formula (based on sex, weight, and age of the patient) may be used to convert this value into creatinine clearance. The serum creatinine should represent a steady state of renal function.

$$\text{Males: } \frac{\text{Weight (kg)} \times (140 - \text{age})}{72 \times \text{serum creatinine (mg/100 mL)}}$$

Females: 0.85 x above value

In patients undergoing hemodialysis, the loading dose of 1 to 2 grams should be given after each hemodialysis, and the maintenance dose should be given as indicated in Table 2.

Antibiotic therapy for group A beta-hemolytic streptococcal infections should be maintained for at least 10 days to guard against the risk of rheumatic fever or glomerulonephritis. In staphylococcal and other infections involving a collection of pus, surgical drainage should be carried out where indicated.

The recommended dosage of MEFOXIN **for uncomplicated gonorrhea** is 2 grams intramuscularly, with 1 gram of BENEMID† (Probenecid) given by mouth at the same time or up to ½ hour before MEFOXIN.

Infants and Children

The recommended dosage in children three months of age and older is 80 to 160 mg/kg of body weight per day divided into four to six equal doses. The higher dosages should be used for more severe or serious infections. The total daily dosage should not exceed 12 grams.

At this time no recommendation is made for children from birth to three months of age (see PRECAUTIONS).

In children with renal insufficiency the dosage and frequency of dosage should be modified consistent with the recommendations for adults (see Table 2).

PREVENTION

General

For prophylactic use in surgery, the following doses are recommended:

Adults:

(1) 2 grams administered intravenously or intramuscularly just prior to surgery (approximately one-half to one hour before the initial incision).

(2) 2 grams every 6 hours after the first dose for no more than 24 hours (continued for 72 hours after prosthetic arthroplasty).

Children (3 months and older):

30 to 40 mg/kg doses may be given at the times designated above.

Obstetric-Gynecologic

For prophylactic use in vaginal hysterectomy, a single 2.0 gram dose administered intramuscularly one-half to one hour prior to surgery is recommended.

For patients undergoing cesarean section, a single 2.0 gram dose should be administered intravenously as soon as the umbilical cord is clamped. A 3-dose regimen may be more effective than a single dose regimen in preventing postoperative infection (esp. endometritis) following cesarean section. Such a regimen would consist of 2.0 grams given intravenously as soon as the umbilical cord is clamped, followed by 2.0 grams 4 and 8 hours after the initial dose.

Transurethral prostatectomy patients:

One gram administered just prior to surgery; 1 gram every 8 hours for up to five days.

PREPARATION OF SOLUTION

Table 3 is provided for convenience in constituting MEFOXIN for both intravenous and intramuscular administration.

For intravenous use, 1 gram should be constituted with at least 10 mL of Sterile Water for Injection, and 2 grams, with 10 or 20 mL. The 10 gram bulk package should be constituted with 43 or 93 mL of Sterile Water for Injection or any of the solutions listed under the *Intravenous* portion of the COMPATIBILITY AND STABILITY section. CAUTION: THE 10 GRAM BULK STOCK SOLUTION IS NOT FOR DIRECT INFUSION. One or 2 grams of MEFOXIN for infusion may be constituted with 50 or 100 mL of 0.9 percent Sodium Chloride Injection, 5 percent or 10 percent Dextrose Injection, or any of the solutions listed under the *Intravenous* portion of the COMPATIBILITY AND STABILITY section.

Benzyl alcohol as a preservative has been associated with toxicity in neonates. While toxicity has not been demonstrated in infants greater than three months of age, in whom use of MEFOXIN may be indicated, small infants in this age range may also be at risk for benzyl alcohol toxicity. Therefore, diluent containing benzyl alcohol should not be used when MEFOXIN is constituted for administration to infants.

For ADD-Vantage® ††† vials, see separate INSTRUCTIONS FOR USE OF MEFOXIN IN ADD-Vantage® VIALS. MEFOXIN in ADD-Vantage® vials should be constituted with ADD-Vantage® diluent containers containing 50 mL or 100 mL of either 0.9 percent Sodium Chloride Injection or 5 percent Dextrose Injection. MEFOXIN in ADD-Vantage® vials is for IV use only.

For intramuscular use, each gram of MEFOXIN may be constituted with 2 mL of Sterile Water for Injection, *or—*

For intramuscular use ONLY: each gram of MEFOXIN may be constituted with 2 mL of 0.5 percent lidocaine hydrochlo-

†††Registered trademark of Abbott Laboratories, Inc.

Table 1 — Guidelines for Dosage of MEFOXIN

Type of Infection	Daily Dosage	Frequency and Route
Uncomplicated forms+of infections such as pneumonia, urinary tract infection, cutaneous infection	3 - 4 grams	1 gram every 6 - 8 hours IV or IM
Moderately severe or severe infections	6 - 8 grams	1 gram every 4 hours *or* 2 grams every 6 - 8 hours IV
Infections commonly needing antibiotics in higher dosage (e.g., gas gangrene)	12 grams	2 grams every 4 hours *or* 3 grams every 6 hours IV

+Including patients in whom bacteremia is absent or unlikely.

Table 2 — Maintenance Dosage of MEFOXIN in Adults with Reduced Renal Function

Renal Function	Creatinine Clearance (mL/min)	Dose (grams)	Frequency
Mild impairment	50 - 30	1 - 2	every 8 - 12 hours
Moderate impairment	29 - 10	1 - 2	every 12 - 24 hours
Severe impairment	9 - 5	0.5 - 1	every 12 - 24 hours
Essentially no function	<5	0.5 - 1	every 24 - 48 hours

Table 3 — Preparation of Solution

Strength	Amount of Diluent to be Added (mL)++	Approximate Withdrawable Volume (mL)	Approximate Average Concentration (mg/mL)
1 gram Vial	2 (Intramuscular)	2.5	400
2 gram Vial	4 (Intramuscular)	5	400
1 gram Vial	10 (IV)	10.5	95
2 gram Vial	10 or 20 (IV)	11.1 or 21.0	180 or 95
1 gram Infusion Bottle	50 or 100 (IV)	50 or 100	20 or 10
2 gram Infusion Bottle	50 or 100 (IV)	50 or 100	40 or 20
10 gram Bulk	43 or 93 (IV)	49 or 98.5	200 or 100

++Shake to dissolve and let stand until clear.

ride solution‡ (without epinephrine) to minimize the discomfort of intramuscular injection.

ADMINISTRATION

MEFOXIN may be administered intravenously or intramuscularly after constitution.

Parenteral drug products should be inspected visually for particulate matter and discoloration prior to administration whenever solution and container permit.

Intravenous Administration

The intravenous route is preferable for patients with bacteremia, bacterial septicemia, or other severe or life-threatening infections, or for patients who may be poor risks because of lowered resistance resulting from such debilitating conditions as malnutrition, trauma, surgery, diabetes, heart failure, or malignancy, particularly if shock is present or impending.

For intermittent intravenous administration, a solution containing 1 gram or 2 grams in 10 mL of Sterile Water for Injection can be injected over a period of three to five minutes. Using an infusion system, it may also be given over a longer period of time through the tubing system by which the patient may be receiving other intravenous solutions. However, during infusion of the solution containing MEFOXIN, it is advisable to temporarily discontinue administration of any other solutions at the same site.

For the administration of higher doses by continuous intravenous infusion, a solution of MEFOXIN may be added to an intravenous bottle containing 5 percent Dextrose Injection, 0.9 percent Sodium Chloride Injection, 5 percent Dextrose and 0.9 percent Sodium Chloride Injection, or 5 percent Dextrose Injection with 0.02 percent sodium bicarbonate solution. BUTTERFLY††† or scalp vein-type needles are preferred for this type of infusion.

Solutions of MEFOXIN, like those of most beta-lactam antibiotics, should not be added to aminoglycoside solutions (e.g., gentamicin sulfate, tobramycin sulfate, amikacin sulfate) because of potential interaction. However, MEFOXIN and aminoglycosides may be administered separately to the same patient.

Intramuscular Administration

As with all intramuscular preparations, MEFOXIN should be injected well within the body of a relatively large muscle such as the upper outer quadrant of the buttock (i.e., gluteus maximus); aspiration is necessary to avoid inadvertent injection into a blood vessel.

COMPATIBILITY AND STABILITY

Intravenous

MEFOXIN, as supplied in vials or the bulk package and constituted to 1 gram/10 mL with Sterile Water for Injection, Bacteriostatic Water for Injection, (see PREPARATION OF SOLUTION), 0.9 percent Sodium Chloride Injection, or 5 percent Dextrose Injection, maintains satisfactory potency for 24 hours at room temperature, for one week under refrigeration (below 5°C), and for at least 30 weeks in the frozen state.

These primary solutions may be further diluted in 50 to 1000 mL of the following solutions and maintain potency for 24 hours at room temperature and at least 48 hours under refrigeration:

Sterile Water for Injection‡‡
0.9 percent Sodium Chloride Injection
5 percent or 10 percent Dextrose Injection‡‡
5 percent Dextrose and 0.9 percent Sodium Chloride Injection
5 percent Dextrose Injection with 0.02 percent Sodium Bicarbonate solution
5 percent Dextrose Injection with 0.2 percent or 0.45 percent saline solution
Ringer's Injection
Lactated Ringer's Injection‡‡
5 percent Dextrose in Lactated Ringer's Injection‡‡
5 percent or 10 percent invert sugar in water
10 percent invert sugar in saline solution
5 percent Sodium Bicarbonate Injection
Neut (sodium bicarbonate)†††‡‡
M/6 sodium lactate solution
NORMOSOL-M in D5-W†††‡‡
IONOSOL B w/Dextrose 5 percent†††‡‡
POLYONIC M 56 in 5 percent Dextrose‡‡‡
Mannitol 5% and 2.5%
Mannitol 10%‡‡
ISOLYTE§ E
ISOLYTE§ E with 5% Dextrose

MEFOXIN, as supplied in infusion bottles and constituted with 50 to 100 mL of 0.9 percent Sodium Chloride Injection, or 5 percent or 10 percent Dextrose Injection, maintains satisfactory potency for 24 hours at room temperature or for 1 week under refrigeration (below 5°C).

MEFOXIN is supplied in single dose ADD-Vantage® vials and should be prepared as directed in the accompanying INSTRUCTIONS FOR USE OF MEFOXIN IN ADD-Vantage® VIALS using ADD-Vantage® diluent containers containing 50 mL or 100 mL of either 0.9 percent Sodium Chloride Injection or 5 percent Dextrose Injection. When prepared with either of these diluents, MEFOXIN maintains satisfactory potency for 24 hours at room temperature.

Limited studies with solutions of MEFOXIN in 0.9 percent Sodium Chloride Injection, Lactated Ringer's Injection, and 5 percent Dextrose Injection in VIAFLEX§§ intravenous bags show stability for 24 hours at room temperature, 48 hours under refrigeration or 26 weeks in the frozen state and 24 hours at room temperature thereafter. Also, solutions of MEFOXIN in 0.9 percent Sodium Chloride Injection show similar stability in plastic tubing, drip chambers, and volume control devices of common intravenous infusion sets.

After constitution with Sterile Water for Injection and subsequent storage in disposable plastic syringes, MEFOXIN is stable for 24 hours at room temperature and 48 hours under refrigeration.

After the periods mentioned above, any unused solutions or frozen material should be discarded. Do not refreeze.

Intramuscular

MEFOXIN, as constituted with Sterile Water for Injection, Bacteriostatic Water for Injection, or 0.5 percent or 1 percent lidocaine hydrochloride solution (without epinephrine), maintains satisfactory potency for 24 hours at room temperature, for one week under refrigeration (below 5°C), and for at least 30 weeks in the frozen state.

After the periods mentioned above, any unused solutions or frozen material should be discarded. Do not refreeze.

MEFOXIN has also been found compatible when admixed in intravenous infusions with the following:

Heparin 0.1 units/mL at room temperature — 8 hours
Heparin 100 units/mL at room temperature — 24 hours
M.V.I.§§§ concentrate at room temperature 24 hours; under refrigeration 48 hours
BEROCCA|| C-500 at room temperature 24 hours; under refrigeration 48 hours
Insulin in Normal Saline at room temperature 24 hours; under refrigeration 48 hours
Insulin in 10% invert sugar at room temperature 24 hours; under refrigeration 48 hours

HOW SUPPLIED

Sterile MEFOXIN is a dry white to off-white powder supplied in vials and infusion bottles containing cefoxitin sodium as follows:

No. 3356 — 1 gram cefoxitin equivalent
NDC 0006-3356-45 in trays of 25 vials
(6505-01-119-6005, 1 g 25's).

No. 3368 — 1 gram cefoxitin equivalent
NDC 0006-3368-71 in trays of 10 infusion bottles
(6505-01-195-0649, 1 g infusion bottle 10's).

No. 3357 — 2 gram cefoxitin equivalent
NDC 0006-3357-53 in trays of 25 vials
(6505-01-104-6393, 2 g 25's).

No. 3369 — 2 gram cefoxitin equivalent
NDC 0006-3369-73 in trays of 10 infusion bottles
(6505-01-185-2624, 2 g infusion bottle 10's).

No. 3388 — 10 gram cefoxitin equivalent
NDC 0006-3388-67 in trays of 6 bulk bottles
(6505-01-263-0730, 10 g 6's).

No. 3548 — 1 gram cefoxitin equivalent
NDC 0006-3548-45 in trays of 25 ADD-Vantage® vials
(6505-01-262-9509, 1 g ADD-Vantage® 25's).

No. 3549 — 2 gram cefoxitin equivalent
NDC 0006-3549-53 in trays of 25 ADD-Vantage® vials
(6505-01-263-4531, 2 g ADD-Vantage® 25's).

Special storage instructions

MEFOXIN in the dry state should be stored below 30°C. Avoid exposure to temperatures above 50°C. The dry material as well as solutions tend to darken, depending on storage conditions; product potency, however, is not adversely affected.

†††Registered trademark of Abbott Laboratories, Inc.
‡See package circular of manufacturer for detailed information concerning contraindications, warnings, precautions, and adverse reactions.
‡‡In these solutions, MEFOXIN has been found to be stable for a period of one week under refrigeration.
‡‡‡Registered trademark of Cutter Laboratories, Inc.
§Registered trademark of American Hospital Supply Corporation.
§§Registered trademark of Baxter International, Inc.
§§§Registered trademark of USV Pharmaceutical Corp.
||Registered trademark of Roche Laboratories.

Dist. by:
MERCK & CO., INC., West Point, PA 19486, USA

Issued March 1994

7882332